ZUMBA®

WITHDRAWN

ZUMBA®

Ditch the Workout, Join the Party!™
The ZUMBA Weight Loss Program

BETO PEREZ

and MAGGIE GREENWOOD-ROBINSON, PhD

WELLNESS
CENTRAL

NEW YORK   BOSTON

ZUMBA®
FITNESS

Copyright © 2009 by Zumba Fitness, LLC
Photography by Justo Pinero

Wellness Central
Hachette Book Group
237 Park Avenue
New York, NY 10017

Visit our website at
www.HachetteBookGroup.com.

www.zumba.com

Wellness Central is an imprint of Grand Central Publishing.

The Wellness Central name and logo are trademarks of Hachette Book Group, Inc.

Printed in the United States of America

First Edition: September 2009

10 9 8 7 6 5 4 3 2

Library of Congress Cataloging-in-Publication Data

Perez, Beto.

Zumba: ditch the workout, join the party! the Zumba weight loss program / Beto Perez ; with Maggie Greenwood-Robinson.—1st ed.

p. cm.

Includes bibliographical references.

ISBN 978-0-446-54612-6

1. Aerobic dancing. 2. Aerobic exercises. 3. Weight loss. I. Greenwood-Robinson, Maggie. II. Title.

RA781.15.P47 2009

613.7'15—dc22   2009006552

To my mother, Maria del Carmen, who is
my strength, and to all the ZUMBA instructors
who wake up every day to make the world
a happier and healthier place.

Contents

Part Three

DITCH BORING DIETS: LET'S EAT TO BURN BELLY FAT AND THIGH FAT 151

Acknowledgments

I would like to thank the wonderful friends and associates who have helped me bring this book together. They are:

Alberto Perlman and Alberto Aghion, the smartest guys I know. I feel blessed that they found me, and then figured out, and executed, a way to take the Zumba philosophy around the world.

Petra Robinson, Koh Herlong, and the talented Zumba education specialists for creating and running the Zumba Academy.

Rodrigo Faerman, Roberto Moreno, Jeffrey Perlman, and Marcelo Borlando for their amazing innovations.

Tania Liberman, Melanie Canevaro, Iliana Soto, Andras Kende, Doug Jarquin, David Perlman, Tessy Staton, Jonathan Perlman, Valery Bronstein, Vanessa Saieh, Barbie Castellon, Michael Chesal, Vicky Zagarra, Esther Benmeleh, Linda Ramos, Deb Orringer, Adele Harrington, Alyson Rodriguez, Miri Aghion, Stephanie Perlman, and the rest of the Zumba office for being so dedicated to providing all the Zumba instructors with everything they need.

Walter Diaz, Hugo Calero, and Marcelo Cezan for being my friends through all the ups and downs.

Maggie Greenwood-Robinson for making me sound smart and putting the words in my heart on every page.

Barbara Lowenstein, my terrific agent, who made this book happen.

Diana Baroni, my editor, and everyone at Grand Central for seeing the power of Zumba and publishing this book.

The many, many people I have met through Zumba. I may not be good at remembering all your names, but I remember your passion and commitment to this fitness movement, and I am grateful for every one of you.

—*Alberto "Beto" Perez*

Part One

DITCH THE WORKOUT, JOIN THE PARTY!

Introduction

WHAT IS ZUMBA?

If you are wondering what Zumba® is, you have come to the right place. The book you are holding in your hands is your guide to the largest, most popular Latin-inspired dance fitness class in the world. Zumba has created an exciting new brand of fitness: a high-energy program with motivating music and dance moves drawn from salsa, merengue, and other Latin steps and free-form styles. It integrates some of the basic principles of aerobic, resistance, and interval training to tone and sculpt your body, burn fat, maximize caloric output, and benefit your heart and mind.

In this book and in the exclusive DVD that accompanies it, you will learn these popular Latin dances so that you can dance your way to a beautiful body in no time. I simplified the steps and put them together so that exercising feels like a dance party. That way, Zumba is easy for anyone, regardless of age or ability. I do not care if you are on your left foot or right foot; I just want you to have fun and get a great workout!

Years ago, I would never have imagined that Zumba fitness programs would become so popular and be made into a book. Back in the 1990s I was teaching aerobics classes at a fitness club. I showed up one day to teach but had forgotten my regular music. I was forced to improvise on the spot! Fortunately, I had some Latin music with me, so I popped those tunes in the tape deck and started doing Latin dances to them. Everyone in the class loved it, and Zumba was born. I have been both humbled and surprised that Zumba took off worldwide from there.

The overwhelming success created a demand for more information on Zumba and how to do it—which is why I wrote this book and created its exclusive companion DVD. Nowhere will you find a more definitive and unique guide to Zumba than right here. I designed this groundbreaking fitness plan specifically for this book. You can use it and the DVD to learn and practice Zumba at your own pace, on your own schedule, right at home—and have a lot of fun while getting into amazing shape.

Now, for the first time ever, you will be introduced to the exclusive Zumba Diet, a unique food plan that focuses on "bodyshaping foods," foods that have been scientifically proven to take fat off your abs, thighs, and all over your body. You will learn how to do this quickly, too, by starting with the Zumba 5-Day Express Diet, which can help you lose up to nine pounds in five days. Then you move on to one of the bodyshaping diets: the Zumba Flat Abs Diet, the Zumba Thin Thighs Diet, or the Zumba Basic Diet, depending on your goals. You will continue to lose weight steadily, too, and could be about twenty pounds lighter in about two months.

I have divided the book into three parts: Part One deals with the origins of Zumba—what it is, how it got started, and what it will do for your body and mind. Part Two gets the party started. You will learn about the music, the steps, my sculpt-and-tone moves, and the Zumba routines. Everything you need to know is clearly described and demonstrated in more than 120 photographs. Do not make the mistake of thinking that a Zumba routine is like other, more monotonous forms of dance exercise. It is not! As you work through this book and watch the DVD, have fun, and work at your pace. If necessary, read through the relevant sections several times until you become totally familiar with the moves.

Finally, Part Three introduces you to the Zumba Diet, so that you start losing weight quickly, reshape your body, and get to your ideal weight. When you combine Zumba with this bodyshaping nutrition program, you can melt pounds away fast—and keep losing fat consistently from there. *Zumba* brings together everything you need to know about the world's most enjoyable way to lose weight and get fit.

Whether you are new to Zumba fitness programs or already a fan, this book will help you derive exceptional health and fitness benefits, all in an atmosphere of fun. If you follow what I have set out for you here, you will experience a dramatic transformation in your physical and mental well-being. For example, you will:

✳ **Burn Hundreds of Calories in an Hour.** Zumba burns a significant number of calories, depending on how much you put into it. Why is Zumba so good at torching calories? It is a form of interval training, in which you increase and decrease the intensity of your workout through varied rhythms and dance styles. Interval training has been shown in research to burn more calories.

✳ **Lose Up to Nine Pounds in Five Days.** Every great workout program needs a great nutrition program to complement it—which is why the Zumba Diet was created. The diet is unique in that it is built around healthy foods that have been scientifically shown to encourage fat loss in your abs, thighs, and all over your body. So while Zumba is burning fat off in places where you do not want it, the Zumba Diet is enhancing that process with its special bodyshaping foods. As I mentioned earlier, you have the option to jump-start the shaping process with the Zumba 5-Day Express Diet, which can take off up to nine pounds in five days—without deprivation, while you eat only healthy, energy-giving foods. Losing a lot of weight right off the bat gives you a psychological boost, too. You will want to keep losing through healthy eating and fun exercise. You simply cannot fail when you combine the Zumba fitness programs with the Zumba Diet.

✳ **Use My Enclosed, Exclusive DVD to Have the Time of Your Life.** I have made it so easy and fun for you to learn Zumba's fitness routines by including a DVD with this book. It features the basic steps and music for the routines outlined in this book. You can study the steps and the routines in the book, then put them into action by following the DVD. Unlike aerobics DVDs, the choreography in Zumba is based on lyrics—you have one set of moves for the chorus and another for the verses. This makes Zumba surprisingly easy to follow.

✳ **See a Real Difference in Your Shape.** Zumba also has its strength-training components. Many of the dance steps incorporate fitness variations like squats or lunges. You can also sculpt your body with some of my special toning moves. So in addition to getting your heart rate up, Zumba works your thighs, butt, core, upper body, and all your trouble spots. Use the Zumba Diet to help this reshaping process along, and see results quickly.

✳ **Enjoy Exercising for the First Time in Your Life.** I know that the wild popularity of Zumba is rooted in the fact that it makes fitness fun. And when something is fun, it is just human nature to come back for more—and to stick with it. When your workout is over, you will be tempted to pop the DVD back in and repeat your exercise session! So if you despise working out, are battling that bulge, or have been ordered to exercise by your doctor, then consider this as a fun way to move toward a healthier you. It is "easy medicine."

✳ **Feel Wonderful.** What is good for your body is usually good for your mind, and Zumba is no exception. The workouts also serve as a stress reliever, a mood lifter, and a confidence builder. You will start feeling better about yourself after you start exercising to the DVD and taking off pounds with the diet.

If all of these benefits are not reason enough to get moving, research shows that people who are in shape, active, and fit live longer than people who are not. That said, don't you think it is time to let Zumba help you melt away the bulges and blues, have fun, and help you get the most out of life?

I would say so. Okay, now I invite you to join me for Zumba!

Chapter 1

WELCOME TO ZUMBA

There is a serious party going on. Pulsating international beats fill the room. People of all sizes and shapes begin to sashay and gyrate to the music, with verve and attitude, shaking their buns and swaying their arms. Soon the room takes on the vibe of a dance club. As I start to lead the Zumba class, I look out at all the faces. I see smiles, I hear laughter, and I feel joy. It is a very humbling experience when I realize that people are happy and having fun while exercising.

It is this fun that keeps them coming back.

What hooks people—even people who do not like to exercise—is that they experience so much happiness while moving to the beat of the music. Yes, Zumba classes are all about joy and fun. You do not need to know how to dance. You do not need to memorize steps. You just have fun. And you get results.

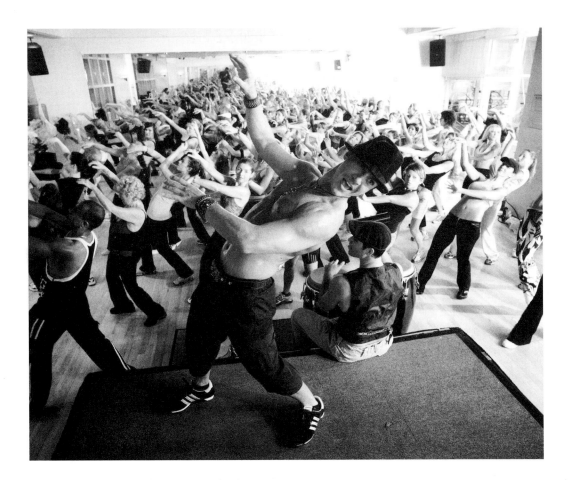

At this point, you are probably thinking, "But, Beto, I hate exercising! I will find any reason in the world—dirty dishes, a bathroom that needs cleaning, phone calls to make—to push it off."

Great—I am glad you admit it. With Zumba, you do not even realize you are exercising because you will be so caught up in the music and movement. In a brief hour of Zumba, you will feel like you are dancing the night away. In fact, the experience is like going to a nightclub and dancing. You will not be thinking about quadriceps or biceps. You will not be counting reps. You will not be looking at your watch. You will not want to stop. You will be having fun in a non-intimidating atmosphere, and you will feel disappointed when your workout ends.

So, what exactly is Zumba (pronounced *ZOOM-bah*)?

DANCE FITNESS AT ITS MOST DYNAMIC

Zumba is the largest Latin-inspired dance fitness brand in the world. It incorporates moves such as the merengue, mambo, salsa, rumba, cha-cha, and others into an amazing workout. All of this happens in a healthy, fun, party-like environment with passionate and explosive music that just makes you want to move. And with the program I have created for this book and its companion DVD, you will be able to duplicate this experience at home.

A WORKOUT THAT BREAKS ALL THE RULES

I like to say that "Zumba breaks all the exercise rules." As a dance-based workout, it is fairly free-form. There is an organized flow to the routines, but you do not have to follow them perfectly. Nor do you have to pay much attention to counts or turns, only to the beat of the music. You just move your body to that beat—or, rather, let the beat move your body. With Zumba, I place emphasis on the importance of each person enjoying his or her experience.

Unlike traditional aerobics, where you often move like a rigid cheerleader jumping up and down or kicking your legs out straight, with Zumba routines you are using your whole body and flowing with the music. This aspect of Zumba lets you whittle your waistline, tone your legs and buns, and sculpt your entire physique.

In the truest sense, Zumba will move you from the inside. It frees your emotions and makes fitness a cut-loose activity. It provides variety and uplifts your spirits. Zumba participants do not say "I should exercise," they say "I can't wait to exercise."

EXERCISE IN DISGUISE

Zumba was born out of my passion for music, dance, rhythms, and fitness. Most important, I felt that workouts needed a huge dose of fun—with party-like, no-thinking elements—to make them appealing to everyone, not just for fit, coordinated folks. I decided to put fun into fitness, and Zumba caught fire. And that is the secret to Zumba's success: It is fun, and it does not feel like exercise—which is why people love it.

Zumba fans come from all walks of life, and they flock to it for many reasons besides the fun factor. People tell me they like Zumba because it makes them forget they are working out. They like Zumba because it is soft and safer on the joints—no pounding or jumping. They join Zumba classes because they are tired of impersonal gyms filled with hulking machinery. They love Zumba because it helps them lose inches and pounds, without the usual discouragement of dieting or the boredom of exercise.

DANCE EXPERIENCE NOT REQUIRED!

You know the feeling: Your favorite music is playing. You may be at your desk, bent over your computer. You may be in the kitchen, whipping up dinner. You may be standing under the shower. Chances are you are tapping your feet and moving to the beat. You are feeling the powerful sway dance holds over us.

From ancient times, humans have danced to express their feelings, to communicate their culture, and to free their spirits. Cavemen did it before the hunt to gain spiritual power from the animals, and ancient Greek soldiers did it as training for battle. There are wedding dances, welcoming dances, fertility dances, rain dances, and spiritual dances. In every era and culture, people have danced to celebrate or commemorate just about anything conceivable. I cannot think of a more universal way to honor our physical existence, or to celebrate life, than with dance. Today, we know that dance has both psychological and physical benefits. Dance can help relax the mind, condition the body, and relieve physical and mental stress.

Dancing is not just for prima ballerinas or music video stars, either. I really believe dance belongs in health clubs as much as it belongs in nightclubs or onstage. As for Zumba, it does not matter if you have never taken a dance class or just stepped off Broadway—anyone can do it. You do not need to know how to dance. You just cut loose and have fun. Best of all, you shed pounds and inches quickly.

Even if you find dance intimidating, I believe you can overcome your fear if you just give Zumba a try. You can do this in the privacy of your own home. Just try the routines here, use the DVD, and follow along. You will learn Zumba in only a few days. Afterward, you might feel like venturing out to a class. Once you join a class, you will see that there is no competition to see who is the best dancer. There is no right or wrong; it is all about keeping your body moving and having a good time. It is all about what you want to achieve personally through your own Zumba experience.

SPICE UP YOUR BODY: THE PHYSIOLOGY OF ZUMBA

Dancing is wonderful exercise, amazingly good for your health and uplifting for your spirit. By the way, have you ever noticed the longevity of famous dancers: Fred Astaire, 88; James Cagney, 87; Arthur Murray, 95; and Gene Kelly, 83? But what exactly does dancing, including Zumba, do for your body? And what does it do for your mind? The great benefits that come about through Zumba are based both in physiology (your body) and psychology (your mind).

Most people, when they experience their first class, cannot believe Zumba works so well and makes them look and feel so great. With Zumba, you will feel more comfortable, flexible, and relaxed in your body, and you will gain the health benefits many exercise classes promise, but do not deliver. Here is a closer look at those benefits.

Cardiovascular Conditioning

Zumba meets the definition of aerobic activity by its prolonged, rhythmic nature and use of large muscle groups. When exercise is "aerobic," this means it helps your heart, lungs, and circulatory system work better. "Aerobic" literally means "with oxygen." While you work out, your muscles demand more oxygen to work efficiently. As you do more exercise, your body responds by increasing the amount of oxygen it delivers to the muscles and heart. Meeting those demands causes your heart rate and breathing to increase. Oxygen is exchanged for carbon dioxide, which is then exhaled. Your body starts to sweat, and you burn calories and fat. Zumba, or any dancing, for that matter, can raise your heartbeat anywhere from 120 to 160 beats per minute, building your heart's strength and endurance.

In addition, aerobic-type exercise like Zumba:

✳ Strengthens your heart muscle.

✳ Improves your resting heart rate (which means your heart pumps more blood with each beat).

✳ Improves your circulation.

✳ Helps clear unhealthy cholesterol buildup.

✳ Shifts your body into a fat-burning mode.

✳ Increases your metabolism (the body's food-to-fuel process).

✳ Helps normalize your blood pressure.

Muscle Conditioning

If you have ever watched *Dancing With the Stars* or *So You Think You Can Dance* and other dance shows, you may have noticed that all the contestants have really great bodies. Whether they are good at ballroom dancing, Latin dance, or funk, they are all well muscled and have very little body fat. You would not be jumping to conclusions to assume dancing can tone your muscles, and Zumba is no different.

Zumba incorporates elements of strength training into its routines. Strength training involves the use of resistance to increase a person's ability to exert or resist force. It encompasses a range of training modalities such as free weights, bands, tubing, and even your own body weight. The goal of strength training is to condition, develop, preserve, and strengthen your muscles.

Your muscles are the engines of your body. They help drive your metabolism, the body's food-to-fuel process. The more muscle you develop, the faster your metabolism will work and, ultimately, the more calories you will burn. In other words, you burn a lot more calories with a strong eight-cylinder engine than with a weak two-cylinder engine. With strength training, you lose fat faster and keep the weight off because you have bigger and better engines.

Muscle is tissue you do not want to lose, either. It keeps you active and youthful. Did you know, for example, that as you get older you may lose as much as five and a half pounds of muscle every ten years unless you do some strength exercises on a regular basis? With less muscle tissue, calories previously used to keep your muscles toned are deposited as fat. Strength training prevents this from happening.

Zumba develops muscles from top to bottom. Because your arms are held up, you get a great shoulder-toning workout. And because Zumba requires some bending and moving in every possible direction, it works many other muscles. There is a lot of lower-body work—specifically in the inner and outer thighs—because we do a lot of crossover steps. People tell me they can feel the workout in their lower bodies, mainly in the hip area, after taking just one class. When you incorporate my special sculpt-and-tone moves into your cardio workout, your muscles will get even stronger and more shapely.

The movements you perform through exercise, sports, and even daily living can put stress on your joints, tendons, and ligaments. Well-conditioned muscles, however, ease this stress by aiding in shock absorption and protecting against impact injuries. Muscle conditioning has other benefits, such as improving your posture, increasing bone density, and reducing body fat.

If you take Zumba classes, toward the end of a class an instructor may guide you through important muscle-conditioning exercises. This might include arm work with some light weights and a "butts and guts" portion during which you might do crunches, bridges, and leg lifts. Eventually, the class ends with some stretching exercises, performed to a slow, Latin-inspired song.

You can do the very same exercises at home, and I will show you how in Chapter 6. There you will find some exciting ways to strengthen, tone, and sculpt your muscles—and do it without heavy weights or complicated exercise machines. My muscle-conditioning workouts are fun, too, since we do them to amazing music. The music motivates you to do the exercises with more intensity (effort) than if you were doing a series of regular squats or a set of controlled lat-pulldown exercises in a noisy, distraction-filled gym.

I incorporate power moves such as moving side squats or traveling lunges as part of the overall choreography and flow of a Zumba routine. I use inexpensive resistance equipment, such as light dumbbells and special toning sticks that sound like maracas when shaken. You can work out to different types of music, perform a particular move in a double-time rhythm, or just add what I call "attitude" to give zip to your steps. More than a mental concept, attitude is implied in the way you move. Adding a hand accent or a special kick or sexy shimmy— these all spice up your moves and give them attitude. Remember, Zumba is all about breaking loose and having fun.

Core Strength

If there is one thing most people want, particularly during the summer months, it is a tight, toned midsection (core) to show off in bathing suits and bikinis. But let me tell you, hundreds of crunches will not cut it for long. A truly effective core workout has several key ingredients: a variety of strength moves, torso-toning cardio, and a fun factor to help you stick with it. Zumba supplies all three ingredients. It works your entire body, but it is exceptional for working the core because of all the twisting moves you will do and the high control of your torso that Zumba requires.

Core strength is essential to developing a beautiful, buff body from head to toe.

Think about it: All movement comes from your center. If your center is not strong, the rest of your body is not going to be strong, either. Zumba naturally works the muscles that help keep your belly flat and firm, and those stabilizing muscles that support your torso and help you stand tall.

Higher-intensity exercise (like Zumba) is known to burn abdominal fat quite efficiently. When you exercise aerobically, your body releases hormones that activate the breakdown of fat. Abdominal fat is very responsive to these hormones and is burned more easily than fat elsewhere on the body.

You have probably heard that where you store fat affects your health. People with fat distributed in the abdominal area are more likely to have higher triglyceride levels, high blood pressure, and high blood sugar and are more likely to die of cardiovascular disease at an earlier

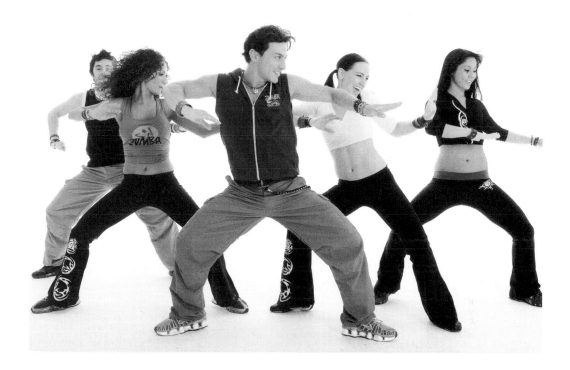

age than individuals who are the same age and weight, but have fat distributed in the lower body. So by whittling your waist, you are not only creating better curves, you are building better health.

Also, a strong core:

✳ Improves your posture.

✳ Gives you a healthy, limber spine.

✳ Provides better balance.

✳ Helps you walk taller (which makes you look slimmer).

✳ Increases agility and flexibility.

✳ Makes you less susceptible to many accidental and overuse injuries.

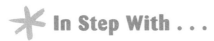 **In Step With . . .**

Debi Baughman, La Porte, Indiana

Debi's story begins with these words: "Zumba was instrumental in helping me rebound from a debilitating health condition. At forty-eight years old, I am healthier and stronger than I have ever been."

In 1973, Debi was diagnosed with scoliosis, at age thirteen, and wore a body brace for three years to stabilize her spine and prevent increased curvature. She was released from her orthopedic surgeon's care in 1978 and did not give her scoliosis a second thought. "As far as I was concerned, I was cured!"

But in 2004, Debi began to struggle with chronic back pain. She had difficulty standing for periods longer than forty-five minutes. Her back would stiffen up. Incapacitating pain throbbed through her lower back and hips. The pain became her constant companion, interfering with her daily activities, both at work and at home.

"Simple things like cooking, cleaning, grocery shopping, were tasks I found nearly impossible to complete. At night, I was often unable to sleep due to excruciating back and hip pain. My chronic pain left me feeling very discouraged. I couldn't help but wonder if I was in this much pain at age forty-four, what did my future hold?"

Debi researched her condition and connected with a physiatrist, a physician who specializes in rehabilitation, whose clinic was 150 miles from her home. Extensive diagnostic testing revealed a 30-degree curve in her lumbar spine and a leg length discrepancy of 1.3 cm. "My scoliosis was much worse than it was when diagnosed in high school. The physician prescribed a course of physical therapy that concentrated on core strengthening exercises."

To further help her condition, Debi was introduced to Zumba and its core-strengthening benefits.

After only eight classes, Debi was amazed at how much stronger she had become. "My back and hip pain had decreased significantly; I was sleeping well, and my lower body started feeling better. Zumba has had such a positive impact on my physical health and well-being. It's really amazing."

Fat-Burning

After Zumba took off worldwide, something else happened along the way, something phe-nomenal. People kept telling me not only how much fun they were having in Zumba, but how much weight they were losing—fifteen pounds, twenty-five pounds, fifty pounds, all the way up to 100 pounds! A fitness movement that was meant to put fun into exercise was taking fat off like crazy.

So just how good a fat-burning fitness program is Zumba?

Zumba uses up energy in the form of calories. To burn enough calories to shed body fat, you must up your activity level, and there are a variety of ways to do it, including Zumba. Obviously, the more exercise you do, the more calories you will expend. The beauty of Zumba is its high calorie burn. You can burn up to 600 to 1,000 calories an hour, depending on whether you dance delicately or work it until you are dripping like you just came out of the pool.

You can lose quite a bit of body fat if Zumba is a regular part of your fitness program. One pound of body fat contains about 3,500 calories. Let's say you gradually built up to doing the Zumba program three times a week for an hour each time; you would burn nearly 12,000 calories in one month—almost 3½ pounds of body fat. In a year, that's forty-two pounds!

Why does Zumba's brand of exercise burn so many calories? It combines not only aerobic training and muscle toning, but also "interval training." Basically, interval training alternates short bursts of higher-intensity exercise with intervals of slower activity that allow the body a break. Interval training releases hormones that create lean muscle, burn calories and fat, and work neglected muscle fibers. Interval training is like adding mountains and valleys to a workout. These "intervals" mimic real life. If you have ever been late for a flight and had to rush through an airport while carrying luggage, you have probably felt the mountains and valleys of life's interval exercise demands. There are a number of advantages to exercising in intervals, but one of the prime payoffs is a higher calorie burn per workout than most forms of exercising. Studies also show that fat loss is nine times greater with this type of training than moderate-but-steady forms of exercising (like walking on a treadmill for forty-five minutes). So by doing the Zumba program, your body will burn fat like nobody's business.

As I mentioned earlier, Zumba can also help boost your metabolic rate. This means your body breaks down stored fat and carbohydrate for energy faster than if you did not exercise. With Zumba, you will be adding attractive muscle to your body. Muscle burns fat. A pound of muscle requires at least thirty-five calories a day to function; a pound of fat needs only one or two calories. So when you build muscle, your body is burning more calories—which means fat is melting away—even when you are asleep or resting. So the bottom line is that Zumba gets your muscles moving and your heart pumping—two actions that force your body to start breaking down fat for energy.

One more important point regarding fat-burning: As fitness professionals, we have done a relatively good job of helping people lose weight, but we have not been successful in helping them keep it off. This is the problem on which we need to focus. Fortunately, regular exercise helps you keep weight off after you have lost it. The key is to stick to your exercise program. That is easy with Zumba.

Flexibility

Can you touch your toes without feeling pain? Reach an overhead cabinet without trouble? How about pulling weeds and not getting sore the next day? If so, your body is flexible. Flexibility is the range of motion around a joint. It can be developed with a program of regular stretching.

At the conclusion of a Zumba workout, you will do some stretches to help improve your flexibility. The tissues in our body—muscles, ligaments, and joints—are like rubber bands. The more you stretch them, the more elastic they become. When you consistently stretch after your workouts, your muscle and joint range of motion will increase. Basically, you will become more limber and agile.

Flexibility also:

✳ Gives your muscles a more elongated look while improving posture.

✳ Soothes sore, tight muscles.

✳ Reduces the risk of injury.

✳ Makes you feel more youthful.

✳ Reduces low back pain.

✳ Helps you better perform day-to-day activities (what fitness professionals call "functional fitness").

✳ Relaxes your body and mind.

A HEAD-TO-TOE TRANSFORMATION

Zumba is a total-body workout. You do a lot of multi-muscle moves, such as lunging while using your arms, pressing a light weight, or doing a biceps curl while squatting. Also, when you work your arms and legs simultaneously, you are using your core muscles as stabilizers, so your abs gets worked without having to do sit-ups!

While Zumba works every major muscle group, it is not like any other exercise routine. As dance, Zumba surprises your body with new activities, helping it to work harder. It promotes individual expression, coordination, and awareness of body alignment. You do not have to struggle to follow combination steps or transitions, but instead you can concentrate on naturally moving your body in new and different ways. By using previously untrained specific muscles, Zumba adds curvaceous definition to your body—a perk I am sure you will love.

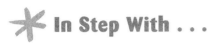
In Step With . . .

Lois Huyghue, St. Petersburg, Florida

Sometimes a miracle emerges from the darkest hours of life. Meet "miracle woman" Lois Huyghue. She suffered a stroke at eighteen months old that left her paralyzed on the left side of her body. The first time Lois saw a Zumba Fitness DVD, she fell in love with its music and rhythms. But she did not know if she could master it, due to her disability.

"I went to my first class anyway. I knew that to learn or semi-master the steps, I would have to really try and practice very hard," she says. "The steps I couldn't get in class I would practice at home."

Lois persevered. It paid off. She was asked to participate in Zumba demonstrations and invited to be on the Tampa Bay performance team. "These opportunities all made me more confident because I had never taught any type of dance class in my life. I was nervous and concerned that my students would focus on my visible disability and not enjoy or even come back to class. To my surprise, they came back and continued coming. At the beginning of my class, I tell them that my left arm doesn't always move in sync with my right one. When I do arm movements, I tell them to use both arms, not just one."

The even more remarkable part of this story is that Lois has since begun to regain some mobility in her left arm. It's hard to say exactly what caused such a stellar improvement, but her doctor is stunned. Lois explains it this way: "I think Zumba has a magic potion inside of the dance that allows you to have more mobility."

Lois has found a calling, too: she serves as a role model to others who are physically challenged. For example, she recently inspired a mother to enroll her disabled child in a Zumba class. "The mother came to me and stated that she would never have thought her child could dance, but after seeing my visible disability, she was determined to bring the child to class and encourage her to do what she could. Already, the mother has noticed more mobility in her child."

Lois performed in a Zumba demonstration at a high school where there were several disabled students in the audience. After watching Lois, they decided to give Zumba a try. And in one of her classes, Lois has a former stroke patient who can now move her left side more than ever. She no longer has to use a cane.

"She told me that her doctor is very pleased with her progress, and she told him it was from Zumba making her force those tight muscles to move. She told me and the entire class that her self-esteem has grown. She feels so much better about herself and is not so self-conscious about the appearance of her arm and leg," Lois says.

There's more to the miracle: This woman is practicing to become a Zumba Fitness instructor. Lois adds, "She now volunteers at the Y and feels like she has a purpose in life."

ENRICH YOUR MIND AND SOUL: THE PSYCHOLOGY OF ZUMBA

When I created Zumba fitness programs, all I did was try to help people enjoy exercise through dance. Little did I know that other benefits would follow. Yes, people were losing weight and toning muscles without even realizing they were working out. But I never dreamed Zumba would become such a transforming force in people's lives. They experience amazing psychological benefits, from enhanced self-esteem to greatly reduced stress. I do not mind telling you that I am humbled beyond words when I hear about such positive changes in people's lives. I admit I do not fully understand it, but I have learned to be comfortable with not knowing all the answers. All I know is that the stories of personal transformation remind me of why I get up every morning to do what I do.

A Brain-Body Connection

Energetic physical movement like dancing activates centers in the brain that pump out happy hormones called endorphins. These natural feel-good chemicals relieve stress, calm anxiety, and lessen depression. They also help keep your appetite under control so you do not overeat. This wonderful body chemistry reduces anxiety and depression.

To prove it, try this quick experiment with me: Just put on your favorite tunes and start to move. Since music is a source of joy, you cannot help but smile and feel good about your life. It is difficult to feel stressed, sad, or angry when you are dancing.

As I like to say, Zumba gives you a triple dose of happiness by speeding up your metabolism, flushing out stress hormones from your body, and increasing levels of feel-good endorphins. Remember, Zumba is dance, undeniably the most universal way of confirming and honoring our physical exis-

✳ **ZUMBA FITNESS TIP:**
Dance Away Dementia

Shake, rattle, and roll—and you just might protect your brain as you get older. A groundbreaking study reported by the *New England Journal of Medicine* a few years ago showed that dancing reduced the risk of various forms of dementia, including Alzheimer's, vascular, and mixed types. The researchers attributed this benefit to the finding that dance is not purely physical; it also requires a lot of mental effort. This shed light on the belief that dancing is a mental exercise as well as a physical one.

tence. I believe that most people need an opportunity to express the power of their being through motion. I know I do. Zumba provides that opportunity.

Motivation

Sometimes you can fall into a rut with your workouts. Your passion for exercise fades and once-exhilarating routines become stale and boring. How can you increase motivation, renew interest, and recharge your energy level? Learn Zumba! With Zumba, you get to that really still place inside of yourself and then the movement flows right out of you. You are not thinking; you are just moving, and you are having fun. You do not want to quit!

You can even add a social aspect to Zumba by using the buddy system. Invite a friend to share experiences and provide encouragement. This can make exercising even more enjoyable—and more motivating.

 In Step With . . .

Danielle Ippolito, Brick, New Jersey

Tragedy is something that enveloped Danielle Ippolito a few years ago. It took Danielle's brother from her and dragged her into a quicksand of depression and self-pity from which she thankfully escaped.

"I never thought I would be okay again," she says. "I couldn't smile for months after. My brother was the greatest light in my life, put out so young. My family is still a wreck and I see how they need therapy over the loss."

As for Danielle, she says Zumba is her therapy. "It is my one-hour session that lets me release all my feelings that build up. I would have never got this if I didn't have Zumba. Because of the support of my class and the people I've met through Zumba, I made it."

Ever since, it has been Danielle's mission to use her example as a way to help others survive tragedy and make it through the tough times of life.

Self-Esteem

Zumba can definitely enhance your self-esteem. It offers a chance to give you positive mental encouragement. Each time you master a step, congratulate yourself. Psych yourself up to try a new move next time. By saying "I can do it," you acknowledge that your goals are within your reach, making it more likely that you will succeed in learning new moves easily. The optimism you develop as a result of Zumba helps you focus on achievement rather than defeat. You will love the way you look in the mirror, too. Appearance is an important element of self-esteem.

 ## In Step With . . .

Debbie Lim-Arena, Farmington Hills, Michigan

Exercise can usually help relieve depression, but Debbie, a group fitness instructor, was not experiencing that relief. For ten years, she suffered from an anxiety disorder and was prescribed medication to help her deal with it.

Debbie confesses that after being in the fitness industry for more than twenty-eight years, the workouts got redundant and she lost her motivation. Along came Zumba.

"I was a skeptic; I've seen many fitness fads come and go," she admits. "But this was different and so much more fun."

Zumba gave Debbie the physical and emotional boost she needed. She testifies that her life has been profoundly changed since teaching Zumba. She is much stronger, more alert, and far more motivated than she has been in a long time.

"I have reached a new level of creative energy and a change of attitude. I am medication free, and I smile more. I can honestly say that Zumba has changed my life."

Stress Reduction

Zumba relieves tension and stress, and improves mood. Because you dance to music in a social setting, you are put in a better frame of mind to work out. You are not as aware of the physical activity because there is so much variety and it is so uplifting. When you catch your groove, there is just nothing that can stop you. It is so freeing. Everyone is happy, and being happy is the best stress cure.

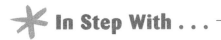 **In Step With . . .**

Doug and Joan Jones, Dayton, Ohio

Late one wintry night in 2002, Joan Jones of Dayton, Ohio, was channel surfing in bed and experiencing the cold Ohio winter blues. An infomercial for Zumba came on and something about the music was magnetizing. Joan, a former personal trainer, ordered the DVDs and taught herself the Zumba steps and routines.

"Even though I never was a very good dancer—I couldn't even do a grapevine step—I absolutely love Zumba. It's addictive."

Joan invited some friends over for Zumba, and pretty soon her at-home classes were ruining the carpet. Joan and her friends moved to a room at the local YMCA, and, after wondering where they could find a Latin guy like Beto to lead them, enlisted her husband, Doug, a bodybuilder and driver for Federal Express, to help lead her growing following.

"I never took an aerobics class in my life before Zumba," Doug said. "I didn't know the difference between a merengue and a salsa." But he got the hang of it and was hooked. During his lunch hour, Doug would often practice new moves in the back of his delivery truck.

"The packages have been cleared out by then, which gives me room to move. But the truck starts shaking. One time the police stopped to find out why. There I was with my shirt off. I didn't want to get my uniform sweaty," he said, laughing.

Joan convinced Doug that they both should teach Zumba. They became one of the first batches of officially licensed Zumba instructors in the country.

"I wasn't used to the idea of teaching a class," Doug said. "Then it started clicking, and I thought, This really is so easy to learn. Now we love Zumba so much that we have the logo tattooed on our bodies."

With no dance background or experience but an instant love for the Latin music and people, the Joneses were able to spread their passion for Zumba throughout Ohio. They are both now Zumba education specialists. The Joneses have also participated in one of Zumba's infomercials.

Eventually, Doug and Joan decided that their Zumba classes needed a stand-alone home. They turned a former shopping center–church sanctuary into a studio with a 1,500-square-foot oak dance floor. With about a dozen instructors and more than forty classes offered each week, the studio brings in hundreds daily to classes and special events.

"We try to create a nightclub experience without the drinking, smoking, and bad pickup lines," Doug explains. "It's great fun!"

Let's Party!

Perhaps you have heard about Zumba but do not know where to begin. Or maybe getting in shape and feeling good about yourself has motivated you to start Zumba. Or perhaps you are already taking some fitness classes but you are ready for something new. I wrote this book to help you achieve all your health and fitness goals, no matter what they are, and do it in a fun, motivating, life-enriching way. If that is what you are looking for, you have come to the right place.

My only rule in Zumba: "Ditch the workout, join the party!"

And it is a party. Read on, and I will tell you the story of how the party got started.

Chapter 2
THE ZUMBA STORY

My dream was always to entertain people. You will find that when you have a dream, you may not always see the way to make it come true; you just have the dream. Maybe you know where you want to go but you do not know how to get there. Do not even worry about it. Just hold on to the dream, keep it alive, and let destiny take its course. This is what happened to me. Perhaps I ought to begin by telling you my story about imagining my dream and then letting destiny do the rest. I will start from the very beginning.

EARLIEST MOMENTS

I came into the world on March 15, 1971, in Cali, the third largest city in Colombia, and was raised there only by my mother, Maria del Carmen. Cali is a cosmopolitan city located in the southwestern part of Colombia. The landscape is mountainous and jungle-like—semi-tropical but not too muggy. The Western Mountain Range of the Andes screens the flow of humidity from the Pacific coast, and we enjoy fresh cross breezes that originate in the west and blow east. The sky has the purest color of blue because the sun is always shining.

The curious thing about my birth is that I almost did not get born at all. When my mother was only sixteen, she fled an abusive stepfather and went to live with her godparents in Cali, where she studied to be a nurse. My mother was, and still is, undeniably lovely. She was not tall, but petite, and had an attractive figure and a lively manner. At age seventeen she met a young man who was training to be a doctor. In those days, as today, Colombian people loved music and they loved to dance. Because Colombia is a country of warmth, people tended to exude a little more sensuality when they dance, and this man was no different. He was a popular, handsome guy whose passion was dance, and he was well known for his talent on the dance floor. Everyone wanted to dance with him. His dancing always brought down the house.

This dashing young man would invite my mom out to the dance rooms in Cali, and so the young doctor-to-be began courting my mother. At seventeen years of age, one is vulnerable. There is no experience, no wisdom, and no maturity. My mother became pregnant with me.

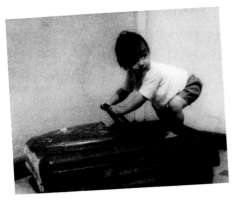

I have always loved cars.

Scared, this man wanted her to have an abortion. This saddened my mother. She also felt ashamed. She decided it would be best to leave her godparents' house and rent a room elsewhere. But her godmother, a woman of considerable strength and compassion, begged my mother to return home, and so she did.

I was delivered healthy, and soon became like a live baby doll, a little toy, for all the other kids in our godparents' household. I was much loved and very happy. Even as an infant I was profoundly stirred and roused by music. I think I was dancing before I was walking.

With a fierce determination and a strong work ethic that would rule her life, my mother decided to get a job as soon as she could to make a better life for us. She became employed by a restaurant, and this meant that I had to be taken to a convent while she worked, since there was no day care in my town in those days. My mother's godmother told me that I went from being a happy, lively baby who was always playing to a very sad infant because the nuns kept me in a crib all day. I was so depressed that I did not eat. The nuns had stern faces framed by stiff white wimples against their black habits. I howled every time I saw a wimple because it scared me so much. One day I developed a fever, and the nuns gave me a cold shower—I was eleven months old at the time—and my fever worsened and I had trouble breathing. The only hospital where my mother could take me happened to be the hospital where my father worked. My father gave me the best treatment possible, and after three days I recovered. He would proudly tell everyone at the hospital, "This is my son." But because my father was married and had two daughters, my mother did not want any contact with him after my illness. That was the last time I ever saw my father.

SCHOOL DAYS

When I was two, my mother and I moved to a one-room apartment in a working-class neighborhood, or barrio, of Cali. The apartments were rough-hewn, box-like structures, stacked on top of each other like building blocks. My mother and I shared precious times of closeness when she came home from work. I played in the dirt streets with other little kids. We had fun and I was very happy.

I was enrolled in school at age four. The first day of school, my mother pointed me in the direction of the school building and told me that I had to go alone. It was a very sad day for both of us, because we would miss each other, and I was frightened, with no idea what life in a school would entail.

Tentatively, I opened the huge doors of the school building and immediately started to cry. For the first time in my life, I felt so lost. I was the youngest and the smallest kid there. A big man, a dark-skinned teacher with black curly hair, reached out to me and kindly helped me find my place in the classroom among the other students. My first day was traumatic, but after that, I was much more relaxed and happy. I should mention that I am left-handed.

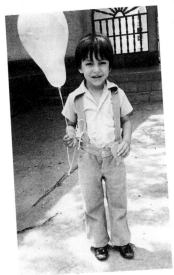

One day we were given pens to learn to write our names. These were the days in Colombian schools when it was considered not good to be left-handed. The teachers bound my left hand so that I would learn to write with my right hand.

I grew up poor, but was happy most of the time, with my mother providing food on the table and love in our home. Not once, living as we did in the barrio, did I see my mom ever falter in her manners or her dignity. Her clothes, though worn and old, were always immaculate and in decent order. She was a kind, tender, always loving presence in my life. And it was my mother who taught me that when you get disappointed you have to look at what you've got and where you're going. Go with the positive things and do not focus on the negative.

Life was fun as a kid.

DIFFERENT HORIZONS

Life grew more promising when my mother met a man named Señor Rios in 1976, and we all moved in together. He had money—bags of money, in fact—and we lived well. We had a driver and we had a boat. Even so, my mother continued to work at the restaurant.

At first I did not have a problem with Señor Rios. He encouraged me to read, and this was good. He would quiz me about what I had read. But if I did not have the right answers, his fury mounted. He would spank me, hard, and threaten me with more spankings if I tattled to my mother. I had never known such panic, so I kept silent. All this was in my sixth year.

Among my earliest memories of this time was the day I drove my little toy cars through a mountain of white sand-like powder that Señor Rios had emptied from a plastic bag onto the table in our living room. Of course I did not know it at the time—I thought I was playing in sand—but the fine white powder was cocaine. Unbeknownst to my mother or me, Señor Rios was in the drug trade.

He became an even bigger figure of fear when I discovered he was hitting my mother. Her eye blackened, her face contorted with disgust, and, weeping uncontrollably, she could not tell me what had happened, but I knew. The intolerable outrage of the abuse made Señor Rios my enemy. I decided to kick him hard, and my kick found a target between his legs. I dashed out of the house for fear that he would shoot me with his gun. I slept in the streets. My young life was in a state of crisis. Consumed with worry for my mother, I returned to the house to rescue her. Señor Rios swore he would never do it again, but the abuse continued. My mother reported him to the police, and he was slapped with a restraining order. He did not obey it. We moved out to escape the violence.

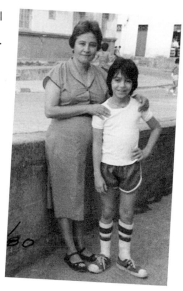

My godmother helped raise me.

DANCE FEVER

One unforgettable day when I was eight years old, my mother took me to see the movie *Grease* starring John Travolta. This magical vision of music and movement awakened something in my blood. Entranced, I knew precisely what I wanted to do: dance! That I was emotionally suited for this profession was not in doubt, for I had a sense of daring and a hunger to entertain.

My mother bought me some Vaseline so I could put grease in my hair and make it look like John Travolta's hair in the movie. Inspired by Travolta's energetic, passionate moves, I began to dance at age eight, mostly at birthday parties. In one month, I became the most popular boy on the block because I impressed all my friends and their parents with my dancing. There was not a birthday party in my barrio to which I wasn't invited. Dance came to me more readily than anything else. The more I danced, the better I got.

I had seen and felt many things that young boys should be spared, and my confidence had suffered as a result. Wisely, my mother enrolled me in judo classes. I loved it. I became a judo champion at age eleven. Judo taught me discipline and gave me self-respect. The wounds of fear inflicted from the years of living with Señor Rios began healing. When wounds heal, they form a scar, which is really good tough tissue, or what my mother called a "thick skin." It gives you confidence enough to go out into the world and to learn to manage the pain of failure so that neither rejection nor defeat devastates you.

My next big dance hero was Michael Jackson. When I was eleven, my mother and I moved into a large home in San Antonio, Colombia, a very nice community. Our job was essentially to house-sit. I had my own room. I would put up a mirror in my room and practice dancing day after day. One day a friend, Ronnie, got his hands on a video of Michael Jackson's *Thriller*. My friends and I were so excited that we left school that day to go to my house and

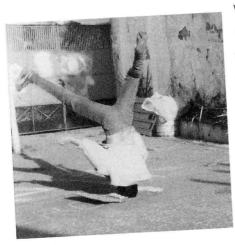

I tried to master as many dance moves as I could—even break dancing.

watch the video. Later, I would watch it over and over again. I learned all of Michael's Jackson's choreography, including the moonwalk, the step where you press into the toe of one foot while lunging and sliding back on the other. You appear to be walking forward while actually traveling backward. As well, I learned the steps of the street, like break dancing, and I could even break-dance on my head. I learned it all.

Music began to drive so much of what I felt in my dancing. When I heard it, when I felt it, I wanted to dance. This is why I tell people that it helps to listen to the music. If you take your time and feel the music, dancing will come more easily to you.

FIRST LOVE

In San Antonio, there was a club for teenagers called Super Cool, an enormously popular spot, open from the afternoon until eight at night on Saturdays. No liquor was served; the club was just for dancing. You could buy sodas to drink, and it cost two dollars to get in. My mother would give me two dollars a week for food at school. For two weeks I did not eat at school in order to save money to go to the club. The first Saturday I could afford it, I packed my good jacket and my white pants in my backpack and off I went to dance. Fearing my mom would not understand my desire to go to the club, I told her instead that I was off to study with friends. Obviously, my mind was not on schoolwork but on dancing only.

I had just one other hurdle: the club's security guard let only the "cool" kids in, so at age thirteen, I had to act cool and look cool. I threw my little shoulders back, I walked with a confident step, and I made eye contact with everyone in my path. As I approached the entrance, I spotted the large cluster of people overflowing onto the road outside. Imagine my amazement when I was allowed to enter. I never felt secure, though, until I had paid my two-dollar admission and was past the guard.

I took the stairs down to the dance floor. A disc jockey was spinning dance music featuring salsa, merengue, and disco, all with driving rhythms and a seductive beat. The music was dense, bright, and hypnotic. There I was in the midst of dancing bodies, flashy turns and breaks, and pounding music, with kids schooled in various Latin dances showing off their expertise and one-upmanship before an appreciative crowd. There was a pure abandonment, a passion. The kids were not afraid to get out there and just go for it. This was like paradise to me. I felt completely free and uninhibited. Everything defied me to stand still. Before I knew it, I was on the dance floor, swaying and feeling the music through my body. The black light glinting on my white pants helped me stand out.

And so every Saturday I went to the club. I grew more confident in my dancing, more relaxed and sure of myself. I had noticed one particular group of dancers who were really good, led by a girl whose name was Sandra, a radiant creature with a mass of soft brown curls falling down around her shoulders. Every curve of her spine, every twist and turn of her hips,

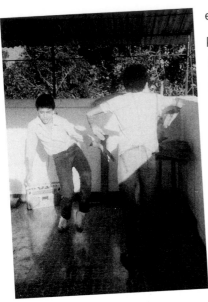

I practiced my dance moves whenever and wherever I could.

every wave of her bangled wrists, was a move from heaven. Power pulsed through her body. No one received more applause than Sandra. She was the best dancer in the club and was always surrounded by guys. From afar I fell in love, not just with her beauty, but also with her dancing ability. I knew I never had a chance, though, because she was in the "cool" group.

One afternoon while I was dancing my heart out, alone, I felt a tap on my shoulder. Wonders of wonders, it was Sandra, inviting me to dance with her. We danced and connected immediately. Every time we danced together, it was like a miniature love story. Incredibly, people fanned out and formed a circle around us when we danced. We had charisma together. She was my first love.

SEPARATION

The world of the dance clubs became my world. I was now dancing at clubs late into the evenings, even though I was only fifteen. It was a time of excitement, wonder, and opportunity, a state of pure bliss, and I lived for the moments when I could dance in the clubs. But for my mother it was a time of worry, frustration, and hand-wringing. One day I found her sobbing in bed and I asked her what was wrong. "I'm worried for you," she said. "You are in the clubs at all hours. I don't want this life for you because it is dangerous." I tried to reassure her that I did not drink, I did not smoke, I did not do drugs, and I was not involved with a bad crowd—that I just loved to dance. But I could not resolve the apprehension she felt for my lifestyle.

My mother was offered an opportunity to go to the U.S., but there was an understandable reluctance. I tried to convince her that she could earn enough money in the United States to buy a house back here in Colombia. I pleaded with her to go until she finally made a deal with me: "If you earn some money, I will go to the U.S.," she told me. Little did she know that I would soon rise to her challenge.

I made several good friends during this time in my life. One of these was a girl who worked at a modeling agency in Cali. She took me to the agency one day and I taught some of the models how to dance. I showed them how to move, remaining loose in the shoulders and upper back, and to sway their hips to the rhythms, exposing them to a diversity of forms and tempos. In fact, I created a whole choreography for them. As the models were going through their routine, in walked the owner of the agency, a serious-looking man named Fernando. He was impressed with what he saw, and the next thing I knew I was choreographing a dance number for the models to perform at an upcoming fashion show at a Cali mall. The fashion show was a huge hit. Never before had anyone seen models who danced. This broke all the rules in the modeling world—as Zumba does in the exercise world. Fernando

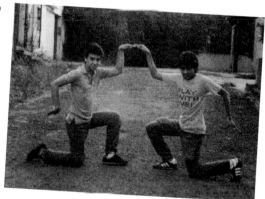

I have always liked to create my own moves; I am constantly experimenting, even if it looks silly.

hired me as an office assistant in the morning and a choreographer in the afternoon.

My first paycheck was thirty dollars. I proudly showed it to my mother, reminding her of her promise. Being a woman of integrity, she kept that promise, and though she was immensely sad, she made preparations to go to the U.S. She boarded a plane to the United States and made her way to Miami, where she gained employment as a housekeeper. I did not see my mother again for ten years.

OPPORTUNITIES

From then on, I lived on my own. At times it was a struggle to survive. I often subsisted on a glass of milk and one banana a day because I was not making enough money at the agency to buy much food. I never shared my condition with my mother, however, because I wanted to prove to her that I could make it alone. I had to grow up and take responsibility for myself and muster up more confidence, all on my own. In the face of this hopelessness, I did the only thing I could: ignore it. I kept my head up, worked slowly and steadily, and did what I believed in. The difficulties inherent in this situation were absorbed by the opportunities to dance. I learned what it means to have something in your life for which you would sacrifice everything.

When I was seventeen, it looked like my big day had come at last. After entering a dance competition, I was selected to represent Colombia at a Latin dance event in Miami. I was so excited because I would be reunited with my mother after two years. I sold everything I owned and spent my savings on costumes. But I never got to compete. My U.S. visa was denied by officials in Bogotá, the capital of Colombia. This was very traumatic for me. I found myself unemployed at the same time.

Then I experienced one of those rare, serendipitous moments of discovery and connection where a lot of good things come together. Earlier, while in Bogotá applying for that visa, I had taken some classes at a local health club. One day, the club owner got in touch with me and told me that one of her regular aerobics instructors was injured. Could I substitute? Although I had never taught an aerobics class in my life, I said, "Yes, I can do it," because I needed the extra cash.

The next day I got hold of a copy of *Jane Fonda's Workout Book* to try to learn something about aerobics. I tried to memorize as much as I could. I struggled to imitate the positions in the Jane Fonda exercise photos. Up in front of the class, I felt awkward at first, and I had to peek at the book's exercise descriptions hidden under my jacket.

Back in Cali, the owner of a gym where I had prepared for my dance routines invited me to teach a children's summer dance class twice a week. I was very grateful to him for giving me the opportunity to earn a living. When I began, there were ten children but the class quickly grew to thirty. I am very energetic and fun-loving when I teach. I try to make my classes as fun as possible, but this is never an act. I think the kids appreciated the authentic energy and laughter I brought to class, and laughter gave them freedom to be who they wanted to be. If I am having fun teaching, I know my students are having fun learning from me.

On the days when I was not teaching my classes, I worked at an ice cream store that served fifty flavors. I loved the job because I love ice cream, and I was allowed to eat it there. On my way to work at the ice cream store, I would pass by the prestigious Maria Sanford Brazilian Dance Academy, where the city's upper class sent their daughters. Sometimes I would glance in the window and watch the instruction—I dreamed of being an instructor there someday—but I was shooed away like a peeping tom, and the curtains were closed. I was not getting paid much and I did not know how to save money. One day, I could no longer afford to pay my rent. So without my boss knowing, I slept for a month in the ice cream store, under the counter. I ate ice cream for breakfast, lunch, and dinner. I know ice cream very well.

It was 1989, and a new dance craze was upon us: the lambada. It began in small Brazilian bars and cafés and remained a genuinely Brazilian expression until a Frenchman introduced the dance to Paris. The lambada took Europe by storm, then spread to the four corners of the world. In the lambada, the couple dances very close together, with their legs seductively intertwined. The name of the dance is a derivative of *lambar*, which in Brazil means "heavy necking." Known as the "forbidden dance," the lambada is danced with the whole body, and usually on the balls of the feet, a holdover from when the lambada was danced barefoot on the beaches of Brazil, where the sand was too hot to step with the entire foot. Naturally, I was eager to master it, so I watched some videos and practiced.

Not long afterward there was a lambada competition in Cali to crown the best lambada dancer in Colombia. For me, competitions were a chance to check out styles from around the country and to improve my own skills. After hearing about the competition, I found myself dizzy with excitement. I grabbed a skilled, experienced dance partner and we entered the competition, which was held in a large, beautiful park in the city. There were more than 1,000 couples competing, and the event was televised by Colombia's biggest television network. We took the competition seriously and we were extremely professional. We danced our hearts out and won! For the first time in my life, I felt important. All of a sudden, the dance clubs in Cali wanted to pay me for performing the lambada on weekends. They would pay me fifty dollars for just one dance. It was easy money, but very good money.

At the same time, my classes at the gym were becoming packed. Every day more and more people attended. Then the most amazing thing happened: the Maria Sanford Brazilian Dance Academy called me. They wanted to hire me, to give me the responsibility of teaching dance classes. I told them they had to give me breakfast and lunch as well as pay me. They agreed, and I happily went to work for the academy.

After I began teaching, I found that a lot of kids were not learning musicality. They did not know how to breathe; they did not know how to feel the music, and so I taught the kids how to interpret the music with their moves. And I would always say, "Do not do this if you don't love it. And if you love it, let me see you love it." And that is what I say to my Zumba instructors today.

Every year, we choreographed a musical. Bringing dance alive in this manner was one of the most rewarding aspects of my work at the academy. My students and I kept pushing the limits of what we could do, demolishing conventions. Our productions made us a cut apart, and in many ways, a cut above, the other classes. One year, for example, we did a musical called *Alcatraz*, a *Jailhouse Rock* hybrid. It was spectacular, slightly edgy, definitely different, and I was breaking all the rules—again.

ZUMBA IS BORN

The academy asked me to teach a toning class in the morning for the mothers of the students. I knew the basics of how to teach it from my experience with the Jane Fonda book—some muscle-strengthening work with some aerobics—and so I started teaching this class on a regular basis.

One day, as I was about to lead my class, I realized I had forgotten my aerobics music tapes. In a panic, I grabbed my own music from my backpack—salsa and merengue from El Gran Combo, Las Chicas del Can, and other popular bands—and told my class, "Today, we are going to do something different," as if I had planned it all along, and I improvised the class for the entire hour. I led the class with salsa, merengue, rumba, and other Latin dances. The effect was electrifying. I could feel the happiness in the air. Everyone started smiling as they exercised. The smiles stayed on their faces long after the class was over. And I discovered that I enjoyed myself deeply, too. It was an enjoyment that came from the gut, a very intuitive response to the music that was full of energy and passion. This desire to make exercise fun has been my philosophy ever since. The joy I found in the participants and in myself forever transformed the way I would teach. I did not exactly know it at the time, but that was the day Zumba was born.

My horizons grew immeasurably at the academy. Not only did I get to teach classes, I was allowed to be a pupil. I was willing and eager, and worked long hours mastering ballet, tap, jazz, and modern dance. Dance, it was my only love. Life was wonderful, and my dreams were coming true, and sometimes accidentally, or so it seemed.

 ## In Step With . . .

Maureen Lewis, New York City, New York

Maureen, a full-time businesswoman in Manhattan and part-time fitness instructor, had never heard of Zumba until a friend at work told her about it and how much fun it was. The idea of a dance fitness class that grooved like a party intrigued Maureen, especially since she had to give up teaching hip-hop after fifteen years because of poor knees. Maureen had never found anything to replace her beloved hip-hop. That all changed after Maureen took her first Zumba class.

"I decided to see what the excitement was all about," she says. "I was hooked instantly, and I fell in love with Zumba the first time I tried it."

The instructor of the Zumba class was impressed by how well Maureen danced and suggested that she become licensed to teach. Maureen followed through, and shortly afterward, she became a Zumba instructor.

"I was thrilled to be dancing again. I now incorporate a little hip-hop into my classes! I'm thankful Beto forgot his aerobic music and improvised the world's first Zumba class. That one day was the beginning of a worldwide phenomenon."

BOGOTÁ

After graduating from the academy, I certainly felt that I was in an artistic infancy, even though I had been dancing and teaching for many years. One thing I discovered was that fresh choreography is constantly in demand. I never liked the idea of doing what everyone else was doing, repeating a choreographic recipe over and over. I liked to renew the creative process each time, and still do. I started earning a name for myself because I would put break dancing and hip-hop in my routines, which was unheard of at the time in Latin American countries.

I was getting a lot of choreography assignments for television commercials in Bogotá, and traveling back and forth all the time between Cali and the capital. Through some friends, I met a Colombian guy named Edgar Gomez, who was studying to be an orthodontist. But he was also preparing for a singing career and auditioning to do an album. A man with long brown hair and green eyes, Edgar asked me to teach him some dance steps to help him in his musical career. So I did, and we became good friends. Edgar went on to become a famous pop star and Latin actor in television and soap operas, but not before changing his name to Marcelo Cezan. I continued to work with this multi-talented man on many of his shows, and was his assistant when he toured. Working with Marcelo was a profound experience for me. Today he is known as the "Ricky Martin of Colombia."

By 1992 I had reached a turning point, and it was time to accelerate the tempo of my life. I was no longer content to keep flying from Cali to Bogotá and back again. It was wearing on me and costing a lot of money, so I decided to move to Bogotá permanently, although I had no permanent job.

I applied for a job as an aerobics instructor at some of the health clubs in Bogotá, but I was at a disadvantage. You see, the most popular fitness instructors in the city were exotic-looking guys, well muscled and sporting waist-length dreadlocks. I was skinny and white. The best I could do was to shorten my name from Alberto to "Beto." I thought at the very least it would sound cool.

I kept pounding on the doors of clubs, hoping for a break. One day, the manager at the Marathon Spa in Bogotá, a woman named Monica, invited me not to teach, but to take classes from their main instructor, Victor. He was good, but undisciplined. After class, he would go outside and smoke cigarettes, and sometimes you could smell alcohol on his breath. Often he just did not show up to teach his class. On one of those days, Monica asked me to step in and teach— another serendipitous turn of events for me.

I got up in front of the class and introduced myself. "I am new in the city, and I am filling in for Victor. He is really a great instructor, and I will try to give you as good as class as he gives you. I do things a little differently, but try to support me, please."

Then I cranked up my music, gave 100 percent to the class, and brought the party up. Everybody loved it. I found out later that the members went to the club manager and asked her to make me the instructor of that class, so I started working at the Marathon Spa on a permanent basis.

During the same period, I was hired by Sony Music to work with some of its singers on their dance moves, artistic expression, and stage presence. I also helped with choreography on two albums by top Colombian singer-songwriter Shakira. It was a happy, exciting time.

MIAMI

In 1995, my mother returned to Colombia, and we were happily reunited after ten years apart. At first, she lived in Bogotá with me, but the climate was too cold for her. We bought our own apartment in Cali, and she moved in there.

A long-running, drug-fueled conflict in Colombia had reached a new peak of violence, prompting an exodus of Colombians headed for Miami. Among them were many of the country's wealthy elite who were some of my best clients in Bogotá. At the same time, I realized I had gone as far as I could in Colombia, and I wanted to take my brand of exercise to Miami.

The first trip I made to Miami was in 1996. I saw the city for the first time through my airplane window, with its ocean-blue waters, massive swath of sand, and pastel-painted art deco buildings. It was a place whose soul is close to Latin America, and I became obsessed with living there. But it would take four trips to Miami over the course of three years before I would settle there. I knew Zumba (which I called Rhumbacize back then) was my destiny; I was not supposed to be doing anything else. During each trip, I went to gyms in South Beach to sell them on my exercise program. But sometimes you go to a place where you know your idea is not welcome because they do not understand it. It is too new. There is an attitude that you come from another planet—you can tell by the funny looks. But I persisted.

Persistence may be the single most important ingredient in starting something new, in facing the fact that not everybody will always like what you have to offer. A few doors may be slammed in your face, for anything new is usually regarded with skepticism at best.

So you learn to put into practice the fine art of persistence. Ask anyone who has ever attained their dream job, and all of them will have something to say about never giving up.

A fulfilling career is more likely for those who persevere. So if you feel blocked or frustrated, gather up your courage, push through it, and keep going. You have to give yourself the chance. You never know what will happen; I certainly didn't. So push forward. It will not always be easy, but you can do it.

Back in Cali, I received a fax from one of the health clubs in Miami, Williams Island Spa, which was frequented by Colombians who knew me from Bogotá. I headed back to Miami, hoping for an audition to teach there, but at first all they gave me were some free passes to take classes.

Another serendipitous coincidence occurred in my life at this time. A friend of mine, Carol, from Bogotá, just happened to be in the gym that day. She begged the manager, whose name was Brenda, to give me an audition. Brenda said, "I'll give you an audition right now."

"Okay, which class?" I asked.

"No class—just an audition in front of me."

Well, it is hard to teach a class and put the energy into it when your class is a class of one. Nonetheless, I agreed.

The room of the audition had big windows, and curious clients started peering through the glass. Assuming a class was going on, they started filing into the room and following along. I brought to the audition the sum total of everything I had been doing in dance fitness. Before long, I had finished my audition with twelve people in the room. I felt like Forrest Gump when he started running and people followed him. I started dancing and people followed me. The class/audition was something of a personal triumph. People raved about the class.

Brenda whipped out her calendar and informed me that she wanted me to teach a special class, in which I would formally audition in front of members of the club. If they liked me, the spa would hire me. This offer seemed like a dream come true, but it had a nightmare side to it. The audition would not be held for a month, and I had no financial means or transportation to stay in Miami for four more weeks. In fact, I was scheduled to return to Bogotá in two days. I gulped and agreed to the terms.

Worried and confused, I paced up and down a Miami Beach street. I was a mess. Then again, something unbelievable and completely unexpected happened. There on the street, I ran into a guy I knew from Bogotá—a personal trainer who could only find work in Miami gyms cleaning the machines. My eyes nearly popped out of my head.

I explained my situation to him. We decided to pool what little money we had and hastily made plans to rent a cheap, tiny townhouse in Little Havana, and buy a used car. We would live in two cubicles of rooms, just big enough for a tiny cot and a chair. Life would be quite spartan. I returned to Bogotá to get my things in order.

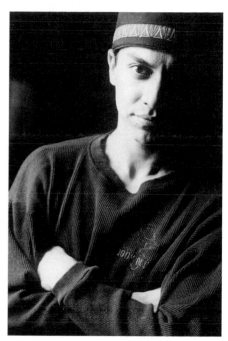

Weeks later, I arrived back in Miami two days before my audition, packing little more than a passion for my program and faith that I would bring it to the US. My friend picked me up in the car we now jointly owned, a 1983 Pontiac with no air-conditioning. Wow, I could not believe that I actually owned another car. I had scrimped for fifteen years to be able to buy one in Colombia; I came to America and bought one practically right away. I took this as an omen of good things to come.

But I almost missed my big audition. Streets were being painted and blocked off. Traffic was crazy. We got lost. Then another miracle: I saw the husband of one of my students in Bogotá right there on the street. He gave us directions.

My first publicity shot!

I arrived ten minutes late. Of course, people in the class were fuming. I silently prayed. Then I turned on my music and just let go. Magically, their emotions changed. They were happy and smiling. All was forgotten. I got in amongst the class, dancing one-on-one with those learning to follow my steps, to encourage them. I did the opposite of what people expected. I danced with the most introverted, the most timid, and the least confident. The students, a mix of women and men, burst into applause when the class was over. They rushed up to me to find out what days I was scheduled to teach. Everything I had done up to this point seemed worth it. I was hired. Soon I was being signed up at gyms all over Miami.

In Step With . . .

Marita Warren, Norfolk, Virginia

Marita often watches with pleasure as her young daughter, sitting in her wheelchair, moves her arms in time with her Zumba Fitness DVD. "I started working out with the DVD, and she fell in love with it," she says. "She loves it so much that I play it for her every single day, at least four times a day."

Her daughter cannot talk, but the look on her face tells Marita how happy she is while watching and listening to the DVD.

While her husband is serving overseas, Marita has been using the DVD to lose weight, and she says it is working well. But the best part of all is the joy Zumba brings to her daughter. Marita says she is grateful for Zumba, and that her daughter is Beto's biggest fan. "Thank you, Beto!"

GETTING DOWN TO BUSINESS

Up to this point in my life, many things had come together, thanks to a series of coincidences that can only be described as providential. It was in Miami, however, that these coincidences took perhaps their most extraordinary turn.

One day, a student of mine, a Mrs. Perlman, told me she wanted me to meet with her son, Alberto, to talk about possibly going into business. I had already had two proposals with some wealthy people who were ready to invest in my dance fitness program. Distrustful, though, I had signed nothing.

I agreed to meet with Alberto at a local Starbucks. Alberto was a young entrepreneur, a fellow Colombian, who had been in the Internet business with a childhood friend, Alberto Aghion, a guy who is very good at mapping out business strategies. Bright and intensely focused, Alberto Perlman has the businessperson's habit of speaking articulately and letting his words hang in the air. I was very impressed with him. We hit it off instantly. Alberto asked me if I had any money, to which I replied, "No." I asked him if he had any money, and he said "No." We looked at each other and said, "Great, let's put it together." All of a sudden, I was a businessman, too.

Both men immediately envisioned my dance fitness program as the next sensation in the world of exercise, and they began to secure funding from interested investors. But my program

Zumba Milestones

1991: Beto Perez forgets to bring his aerobics music to a class he was teaching in his native country of Colombia. He grabs the tapes he had in his backpack, which were songs he loved, as well as the traditional Latin salsa and merengue music on which he'd been raised. Those in the class enjoy the new format so much that they tell him to stop bringing along the other music—and Zumba is born.

2001: Alberto Perlman and Alberto Aghion "find" Beto and together they launch a company, initially built around sales of instructional videos.

2002: Zumba launches via infomercial on national television. The phones ring off the hook.

The first Zumba Fitness Festival is held at the Fontainebleau Hilton, on November 30, in Miami Beach.

2003: People buying the Zumba videos want to learn how to teach it, so Zumba holds its first instructor training workshop. Expecting no more than thirty people to show up, the company is surprised when attendance at the two-day workshop peaks at 150 people.

Zumba partners with Kellogg Company to launch a three-year Zumbando con Kellogg's program that would give away Zumba fitness videos in a promotion on Special K boxes.

2004: Zumba produces the Spanish-language infomercial, sold in thirty countries.

2005: The demand for Zumba instructors across the nation and abroad spurs the creation of Zumba's Educational Division.

Zumba hires an all-star management team including Petra Robinson, former VP of the American Fitness and Aerobics Association; Koh Herlong, fitness veteran; and Rodrigo Faerman, as chief information officer.

2006: Zumba Fitness, LLC, hosts its First Annual "United We Dance" Zumbathon honoring the Quality of Life Fund at Brigham and Women's Hospital.

2007: Zumbawear, Zumba's clothing line, is launched with the original fitness cargo pants, fitness halter tops, and many other active-wear innovations.

Zumba Gold, a class for active older adults, is rolled out and explodes in popularity across the U.S.

Zumba launches in Europe and Asia.

2008: The next Zumba infomercial is produced.

Zumbatomic brand for kids is launched.

The Zumba Educational Division rolls out new courses, including Zumba Basics Level 2 and Zumba Toning.

2009: Zumba introduces Aqua Zumba, a Zumba class developed for pool exercise.

needed a snazzier name. Alberto Perlman, who is enormously creative, came up with Zumba—an invented word, a fusion of *samba*, the lively Brazilian dance form, and *rumba*, meaning "party."

The three of us then set a goal to offer Zumba classes, not just in Florida, but all over the world. Our goal looked like a pipe dream, but we were passionate, determined, and hardworking. One thing led to another, and we soon signed a marketing deal with a fitness equipment distributor to create and sell our DVDs via a thirty-minute infomercial on broadcast and cable channels, resulting in the sale of hundreds of thousands of videos to the U.S. market. The overwhelming response created a demand for Zumba instructors, so we created an instructor training program, with workshops worldwide. The program was an instant success. From zero in 2003, there are now more than 30,000 licensed instructors—and the number is growing. Looking back, it is amazing how far a big goal and passionate dedication can take you.

It was not long before Zumba really started taking off by expanding in more than thirty-five countries through infomercials, DVDs, and major partnerships. Millions of DVDs have been sold, and each week tens of thousands of classes are taught around the world.

All of this surprising success inspired me to write a book so that I could bring Zumba to even more people. Alberto Perlman, Alberto Aghion, and the rest of the Zumba organization also saw the need to offer a nutrition program that would complement the fitness program. And so Zumba Fitness created the Zumba Diet and the Zumba 5-Day Express Diet to give everyone a total fitness package; that is, exercise and diet that work in concert to burn fat and reshape the body. That way, we can help people live a lifestyle that rewards them with a better body, energy, joy, and wonderful health.

Looking back at how opportunities presented themselves, I would not trade my life in dance and fitness for anything. I feel that my happiness comes from the joy and fulfillment of my classes and my students—that is why I breathe; that is why I do what I do.

Which brings me back to the beginning of my story. Seeing something in your mind and actually bringing it to fruition might possibly be the single most fulfilling, satisfying, and truly remarkable process you can experience—especially if the outcome is better than you had imagined. Decide what your dreams are telling you, and use them as inspiration to shape and achieve your destiny. Everything you want in your life is possible.

Part Two
LET'S GET THE PARTY STARTED

Chapter 3

THE ZUMBA WORKOUT: GETTING STARTED

Whether you are brand-new to Zumba's sizzling moves or have taken classes at your local health club, you will find Zumba to be like no other fitness system out there. That is because I designed Zumba, with its scorching fusion of world music and spicy dance rhythms, to make you feel like you are at a party or a dance club. Remember, with its nonstop, easy-to-follow choreography, you can torch 600 to 1,000 calories an hour—*that's a fifth of a pound or more*—and tone your body from head to toe, all without feeling like you are working out at all!

I know that if exercise is fun and easy to do, you will stick with it. And staying with it, making it an integral part of your life, is the key to weight control and long-term wonderful health. Dynamic, exciting, and full of Latin and exotic music flavors, Zumba routines feature aerobic interval training (combining fast and slow rhythms) with a combination of moves that tone and sculpt the body. Zumba targets areas such as glutes, legs, arms, abdominals, and, the most important muscle in the body, the heart! This mixture of dance and sculpting movements delivers an addictive, high-energy workout that I hope you will want to return to again and again.

You have made a great choice to start Zumba routines. When it comes to your body, if you do not use it, you lose it. And the more you move your parts, the more you get out of them. Your range of motion, flexibility, and strength will increase over time as long as you use your muscles, so it is important to keep your body moving. This is how you stay active and youthful.

Getting started takes only a little bit of knowledge, but plenty of enthusiasm. Here is how to begin on the "right foot."

PICK UP THE RHYTHM OF A NEW LIFESTYLE

If you are a newcomer and have not exercised much in the past, take it slow initially, and do not go beyond your skill or fitness level. For someone with no fitness background, twenty minutes three times a week is a good starting point. Over the next few weeks, try to build up to forty-five to sixty minutes a session at least three times a week. You really have to listen to your body; if you feel energetic and want to do more, go for it!

If you are more physically fit, you probably can do more. You should work at a pace that is just beyond your level of comfort but still allows you to hold a conversation. As with any exercise, warm up and cool down your muscles with stretches to prevent cramps and injury. The routines in this book show you how.

Many people get so hooked on Zumba that they go to classes or work out at home five to six times a week for an hour each time. Zumba is just so much fun that it is hard not to want to do it all the time! Seriously, though, your body does need time to recover. For some people, that means working out every other day; for others, that might mean working out several days in a row, then taking a day or two off. Certainly, if your muscles are very sore, you should take a day off to recover. Set up a schedule that fits your body and your lifestyle.

If you are just starting, do not try to imitate me or your instructor too quickly. Get a checkup from your doctor before you begin any exercise program. And remember, dance, including Zumba, is exercise. People tend to have so much fun dancing that they often do not feel how hard they are working out.

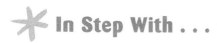 **In Step With . . .**

Neysa Smith, Apollo Beach, Florida

Forty-seven-year-old Neysa Smith, mother of six and grandmother of four, tipped the scales at 193 pounds. It seemed as though every year brought more pounds—and more aches and pains. "My knees and feet hurt every time I stood up," she recalls.

One evening in 2007, Neysa was watching the hit show *Dancing with the Stars*, marveling at how all the stars were able to lose weight from dancing in just six weeks. She had heard about Zumba through an infomercial and ordered some Zumba Fitness DVDs.

"I started exercising with those DVDs and saw a fast change in my overall health and appearance," she says. "Within four months, I went from a size fourteen to a size four and lost forty-eight pounds."

BURN DOWN THE HOUSE!

Not really, but sometimes getting to the gym or health spa sounds easier than it is. More often than we would like, those good intentions may morph into excuses and negative self-talk. When the end of a busy day comes, exercise never entered the picture. For many people, working out at home is the answer—and the solution they prefer.

Many Zumba participants, including lots of our instructors, learned Zumba at home and practiced by watching DVDs. You can do the same, especially with this book as your guide. Here are some suggestions if you would like to start Zumba at home:

✳ Study this book and the DVD that accompanies it. Choreographed with lively, uplifting Latin music, the DVD contains three twenty-minute Zumba routines that incorporate the basic steps and use. Simply follow along and you will be able to master the routines very easily. You can do all three routines in sequence for a sixty-minute fat-melting workout, or do one of the twenty-minute routines, if you prefer. The workouts are very flexible and adaptable to your schedule and fitness level.

✳ Choose a time for Zumba when you will not be disturbed. This might be in the morning, after your kids have gone to school, or in the evening, when you get home from work. Turn on your music, plug in your DVD, shut out the rest of the world—and dance to your heart's content!

✳ Create as much of a home-gym feel as possible by designating a room or an area that is just for your workouts. Make sure this area is well lit and cool enough to allow you to work out comfortably. Equip the room with a stereo and TV. For toning exercises, a strategically placed mirror can help you maintain good form.

✳ Invite a friend or two. If you know a few people who would like to learn with you, gather them together and have your own little Zumba party.

✳ Be consistent. Plan to do Zumba on the same days, at the same times. With consistency, you will see results. And results are the best motivators of all.

SWEAT IN STYLE

There are few hard and fast rules on what to wear. Zumba routines require a lot of movement, so your clothes should be loose and comfortable. Leotards are fine; so are shorts, spandex shorts, cargo pants, baggy pants, and T-shirts. You will be sweating quite a bit, so make sure your exercise clothes keep you feeling cool. Consider clothes designed to pull moisture from your skin, keeping you dry. Polyamide or cotton clothes are good choices, since they absorb perspiration and let your skin breathe. Check out Zumbawear at Zumba.com for some possibilities.

Another consideration is proper athletic support. For women, this means a bra designed for running or aerobics, such as a Jogbra. Men should wear a good athletic support that does not bind.

Good, supportive shoes are a must because your feet will move and land in different ways. These include marching, stepping, lunging, and stomping. Wear sturdy, well-cushioned exercise shoes that are somewhat light but offer good support for your ankles. I am more comfortable wearing lighter-weight shoes because my legs feel more fluid for the dance moves. I suggest an aerobics shoe, a court shoe, or jazz sneakers. Jazz shoes are made to accommodate the rapid directional changes, pivots, and slides that occur in dance-fitness classes. They are also designed to support the foot and ankle while allowing greater flexibility in the ball of the foot and ankle. Running shoes generally have too much tread, which restricts side-to-side movement. Some cross-training shoes might be appropriate as long as they do not have too much tread. I suggest that you go to a shoe store, try on a few types of exercise shoes, and see which one feels the best to you.

STAY HYDRATED

Keep some drinking water close by, because you are going to be sweating a lot while doing Zumba. For best results, I advise drinking plenty of water—between eight and ten large glasses a day. Water is not only the most abundant nutrient in your body (roughly two-thirds of your weight), it is also the most critical. Why? Because it is involved in nearly every process that goes on in your body, from digestion to circulation to excretion. Water, along with other internal fluids, supplies nutrients to nourish body cells and tissues and remove waste products from the body. Water also helps maintain normal body temperature.

Water is indirectly involved in fat-burning, too. The kidneys need ample water to do their job of filtering waste products from the body. If water is in short supply, the kidneys cannot filter properly, so they turn to the liver for help. One of the liver's many responsibilities is mobilizing stored fat for energy. But when it takes over for the kidneys, the liver cannot do its fat-burning job as well. This can stall fat loss.

Try to drink water throughout your day. A good rule of thumb to follow is: Drink a glass or two before you exercise, sip water during exercise, and then have another glass or two after exercise.

ENERGIZE

Zumba routines are a high-energy activity, so you need to fuel yourself properly. Plus, you can enjoy exercising better if you are well fueled and feeling full of energy. If your tank is "empty," exercising could sap your energy.

I have known many exercisers who purposely avoid food for at least three or four hours before exercise. By doing so, they miss out on the performance benefits associated with being well fueled. The "put gas in your car first, then go" theory that works so well for your car also works well for active people. You will have far greater stamina and endurance when you run on fuel, not fumes.

Eating a healthy breakfast of cereal, or toast, eggs, or fruit is a critical fueling strategy. A food combination like this naturally boosts your blood sugar and energy, helping you exercise longer and harder. Consequently, you will burn more calories than if you exercised "on empty." Breakfast also curbs your appetite, so after the workout you will be less likely to reward yourself with high-calorie treats. You will find some great breakfast ideas in Chapter 11.

Another strategy is to have a light snack within an hour prior to doing Zumba to energize you, compared to having eaten nothing. This fueling pattern can really maximize your exercise performance. Good snacks include a piece of fresh fruit, a cup of yogurt, and even an energy bar. I love energy bars, as long as they're low in sugar and low in fat. They are convenient, hassle-free, prewrapped, and portable. More snack suggestions are listed in Chapter 11.

Stay away from snacks and meals that are high in fat, such as bacon, chips, or fast-food breakfasts. High-fat meals will slow you down.

FIND YOUR BREATH AND BREATHE

Breathing is life! Our brain and muscles, along with all of our cells, need oxygen to function. Effectively breathing in (also called inspiration) and out (expiration) not only nourishes the body but increases stamina, mental agility and muscle coordination, and improves range of motion and quality of movement. When I was dancing professionally, I learned that good breath control can mean the difference between an expressive, refined performance and a dull, labored one.

As exercise intensity and range of motion increase, keep your breathing full and draw attention to the working muscles. Increased oxygen uptake will keep you from becoming fatigued. Do not hold your breath while exercising, either, or you could cause significant increases in blood pressure. Hyperventilating or breathing too hard is not a good idea, either. Proper breathing is relaxed and natural.

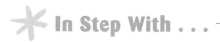

✳ In Step With . . .

Laurel Christensen, Lexington, Kentucky

Laurel was a pack-and-a-half-a-day smoker who detested exercise. "When I started college and had to walk to class, that pretty much covered all my exercise for the day," she says.

A friend who was taking Zumba at a local YMCA encouraged a reluctant Laurel to attend. "I've never been much of a dancer. I've always been really shy and quiet. In fact, I skipped prom, homecoming, and all similar high school functions because I didn't know how to dance and didn't want to be put on the spot. You could say I had two left feet."

Laurel's friend practically forced her to attend Zumba classes, even offering to pay the class fee. "I'd stand in the back and stumble through the steps, lucky to be going in the same direction as the rest of the class. I was so out of shape that I would have to stop for breath early every time."

Her friend became a licensed Zumba instructor and started teaching classes on campus. Laurel attended nearly every one, mostly to give her friend moral support. After a while, Laurel mastered the steps and got hooked on the dancing. "Even though I was by no means fat or overweight, I lost fifteen pounds in the first few months. I had never been more healthy and fit! I even quit smoking!"

After her friend stopped teaching, Laurel dropped out of Zumba classes and went back to her old ways, eating fast food every day and never working out. She drifted back to her old weight and picked up cigarettes again. "I didn't feel as good about myself. When I looked in the mirror, I missed my slimmer figure."

The dissatisfaction with her body renewed her interest in Zumba and she returned to it, doing several workouts a week. Gone for good are all her bad habits.

"If you had asked me three years ago, I never would have dreamed that I would be dancing in public! Zumba has truly changed my life!"

COMPLEMENT ZUMBA WITH
OTHER FORMS OF EXERCISE

The Zumba fitness program is all about freedom. So I say you are free to do other activities along with Zumba. For example, I like to run on the beach, and I like to lift weights.

More people are exploring yoga, martial arts (one of my favorites), Pilates, and an array of different exercises they might not have considered years ago. If you are interested in adding your exercise program, I am all for it. Be open to new fitness opportunities—and ready to act on them—to add to your Zumba experience.

Once a week, celebrate your body outside a Zumba class. Do something just for the fun of it, whether this is a demanding yoga class, riding a bike up a long hill, or going for a strenuous hike—and notice how strong your body is.

DANCE TO YOUR OWN TUNE

I encourage my students to go at their own pace. You should not be working out too lightly nor too intensely. Intensity, or how hard you are exercising, can be gauged by several methods: the talk test, rate of perceived exertion, and heart rate monitoring.

The simplest is the "talk test." It simply means that you exercise so you can carry on a conversation. If you are unable to complete sentences while you are exercising, then you need to slow down.

Another good tool is the rating of perceived exertion (RPE). This 10-point scale lets you subjectively rate your exercise intensity. In other words, you focus on how the exercise feels and learn to listen to your body. Get familiar with how it feels to be at levels 4 through 6 because, depending on your conditioning, that is where I would like you to be exercising most of the time when you do Zumba. Here is the RPE chart:

Perceived Exertion Scale

1 Very easy. You can talk with no effort; this is almost like rest.

2 Easy. This is the way you feel as you move around in daily activities—getting dressed, walking around your office, and so forth.

3 Moderately easy. This is how you feel when walking around from place to place. In addition, this is how you would typically feel during the warm-up and cool-down phases for exercise. Your breathing begins to become elevated, but only slightly.

4 Moderate. You are just below one-half of your max effort, with your breathing becoming more elevated.

5 Moderately hard. This is like taking a brisk walk, or doing a light workout. Your breathing is more elevated. Conversation requires some effort.

6 Still moderately hard. This is how you would feel if you picked up the pace of your brisk walk. Your breathing is deeper, and it is a little harder to carry on a conversation. You feel like you can maintain this level of effort for a while.

7 A little difficult. You have now reached the level of vigorous exercise. Your breathing is quite deep, and your heart is pumping hard. Conversation requires a lot of effort.

8 Difficult. This level feels like very vigorous, very strenuous effort. Your breathing is very deep. It is difficult to carry on a conversation.

9 Very difficult. You are surely pushing yourself at a very high level of effort, and you may start to feel very fatigued. Your breathing is labored, and conversation is impossible. Most elite athletes train at this level.

10 Maximum difficulty. This level requires an all-out intensity that cannot be maintained very long at all. Honestly, there is no value in reaching this level because it can leave you drained and offers no additional aerobic benefits.

The most familiar way to check intensity, of course, is heart rate monitoring. These days, the simplest way to do that is to wear a heart rate monitor while doing Zumba. If you do not have a heart rate monitor, you can check your heart rate in the conventional way, by taking your pulse. Immediately after exercise, find your pulse at the radial artery, located on the thumb side of your wrist when your palm is up. Begin with the count of 1 and count for 10 seconds. Then multiply by 6 to get your heart rate for one minute.

Now, with heart rate, the standard rule of thumb is to estimate your maximum heart rate (MHR). To do this, simply take the number 220 minus your age. Thus, if you are 30 years old, your estimated MHR would be 190.

Many people, and that includes professionals like me in the field, recommend exercising at 55 to 85 percent of your MHR. For the thirty-year-old in my example, that would correspond to a heart rate zone of 104 to 124. At that level of intensity, the body uses a higher percentage of fat calories, compared to carbohydrates, since it relies heavily on fat as a fuel source.

However, if your workout feels too intense, you can decrease intensity by doing slower or smaller foot movements, or by moving your arms but not your feet.

KEEP A RECORD

Expect your body to change for the better once you start doing Zumba on a regular basis. For added motivation, I recommend that you keep simple logs of those changes. The logs should contain start-up information such as body weight and girth measurements.

I believe it is always a good idea to have a specific weight goal in mind prior to beginning a fitness program. In other words, shoot for a weight at which you feel you will look your best. Keep in mind that there is really no such thing as the "perfect" weight because we are all different. There are, however, "healthy weight ranges," and these can be determined through a very simple calculation: Take 100 pounds for the first five feet of your height, and add five pounds for each extra inch to get the midpoint of what should be your ideal body weight range.

If you fall within 10 percent on either side (lower or higher) of that midpoint, you are within an ideal weight range. The lower end of the ranges are for small-boned individuals; the upper end, for larger-boned people. To make this easier for you, here is a chart showing ideal weight ranges (with the midpoints in bold):

HEALTHY WEIGHT RANGES

HEIGHT	WOMEN	MEN
4'10"	81–**90**–99	85–**94**–103
4'11"	86–**95**–105	90–**100**–110
5'	90–**100**–110	95–**106**–117
5'1"	95–**105**–116	101–**112**–123
5'2"	99–**110**–121	106–**118**–130
5'3"	104–**115**–127	112–**124**–136
5'4"	108–**120**–132	117–**130**–143
5'5"	113–**125**–138	122–**136**–150
5'6"	117–**130**–143	128–**142**–156
5'7"	122–**135**–149	133–**148**–163
5'8"	126–**140**–154	139–**154**–169
5'9"	131–**145**–160	144–**160**–176
5'10"	135–**150**–165	149–**166**–183
5'11"	140–**155**–171	155–**172**–189
6'	144–**160**–176	160–**178**–196
6'1"	149–**165**–182	166–**184**–202
6'2"	153–**170**–187	171–**190**–209
6'3"	158–**175**–193	176–**196**–216
6'4"	162–**180**–198	182–**202**–222
6'5"	167–**185**–204	187–**208**–229
6'6"	171–**190**–209	193–**214**–235

Weigh yourself regularly but no more than once a week, and record your weight in a log similar to the one on page 60. More frequent weighing can be misleading and confusing due to fluctuations we all experience from one cause or another. Fluctuations are normal and occur constantly, and they will always appear as a higher reading on the scale when we are retaining water, and a lower reading when we are not. Hormonal changes, degree of hydration, and the amount of salt we eat influence how much water our bodies hold on to. Although it would seem that if you are dehydrated (not drinking enough water), your body weight would be lower, this is not the case. The less water you give yourself, the more the body will be forced to hold on to what it has.

As your weight drops closer to your goal, you will want to monitor your progress in another way, too: by using a simple tape measure and taking "body circumference" measurements, specifically of your abdomen, your thighs, and your hips. That way, you can watch the inches melt away.

Work with a partner and use a simple tape measure to take these measurements. Note whether you measure on the right or left side of your body. If possible, measure directly on the skin, since clothing will affect your values. Take these measurements every three months. Here is what you should measure:

✳ Your waist measurement at your belly button.

✳ Both thighs at their widest points.

✳ Your hips at their widest point. Stand with your feet apart and your abdomen relaxed. Do not take these measurements over your clothes. The tape measure should be snug on your skin, but not constrictive.

Record these numbers and watch them change for the better as you become more fit and shapely with each passing week. Assess your shape in this fashion at least twice—as you begin the program and after you feel you have reached your goal. This assessment provides the benchmark against which you will measure your progress.

WEIGHT MEASUREMENTS

Week 1:	Week 8:	Week 15:	Week 22:
Week 2:	Week 9:	Week 16:	Week 23:
Week 3:	Week 10:	Week 17:	Week 24:
Week 4:	Week 11:	Week 18:	Week 25:
Week 5:	Week 12:	Week 19:	Week 26:
Week 6:	Week 13:	Week 20:	Week 27:
Week 7:	Week 14:	Week 21:	Week 28:

GIRTH MEASUREMENTS

DATE:		
BODY PART	INCHES	RIGHT OR LEFT SIDE
Biceps (widest)		
Chest (widest)		
Waist (narrowest)		
Hips (widest)		
Thigh (widest)		
Calf (widest)		

Of course, we do not necessarily need hard numbers to tell us we are getting fit. The best indicator of progress when it comes to diet and exercise success is the way you look and feel. Do your clothes fit better? Do you have more energy? Do your muscles feel firmer? Are you stronger? Are you able to do things you could not do before? Looser-fitting clothes, increased energy levels, higher self-esteem, and compliments from others often are all we need to know that Zumba is paying off.

DO THE ZUMBA DIET

People are always asking me about diet. As Zumba took off around the world, Zumba Fitness recognized that a sound nutrition plan should be one of the core essentials in our whole philosophy of fitness as fun, diverse, and life-enhancing. We needed a plan that would energize people for exercise, make them feel good, improve health, and help them lose weight. And so the Zumba Diet was developed.

One unique feature of the Zumba Diet is that it is built around "bodyshaping foods" known to help improve your shape, as long as you exercise. Certain foods have been shown in research to take fat off your abs, thighs, and overall body, so naturally you will want to eat more of these foods. The Zumba Diet shows you how, with three diets in one: the Zumba Basic Diet, the Zumba Flat Abs Diet, and the Zumba Thin Thighs Diet. Each plan incorporates bodyshaping foods and includes fourteen days of menus as a guideline.

Consider Zumba Classes

If the thought of spending another hour on the treadmill or stationary bike is enough to drive you crazy, it may be time to look for inspiration from something different, such as a Zumba class. Zumba is fun, no matter if you are home alone or in a group setting. But if you are looking for others who love Zumba as much as you do (and you will, once you get the hang of it and start seeing those results!), then find a class.

Zumba classes are often held at community centers, local YMCAs, health clubs, neighborhood gyms, and dance studios. To find a class near you, call around, or, better yet, look on the Internet at www.zumba.com, then click on "Find a Class" for a list of offerings in your area. Keep checking back, too, since new classes are popping up all the time. A number of classes are geared toward beginners, kids, and older adults. Classes will keep you motivated, help you perfect your technique, and allow you to update your routines and experience new music, too.

Another special feature of the Zumba Diet that makes it unique is the 5-Day Zumba Express Diet, an easy-to-follow diet that lasts only five days and can help you drop up to nine pounds during that time frame. What a terrific way to get started on your way to a more attractive body!

Not only that, the Zumba Diet helps fuel your body with the proper nutrients so you can function at your best. You will eat natural foods that are delicious and nutritious. Strong, healthy people are strong and healthy on the inside because they feed their cells with nutri-

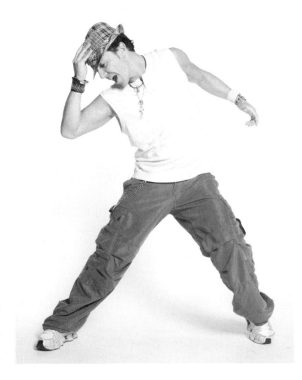

ents that enhance the cells' constitution. When you eat right, you have more mental and physical energy. You will start to look younger, too. And of course you will lose plenty of weight.

I watch my own diet very closely. A few years ago, I did not have to be so vigilant because I was teaching twenty-two classes a week. I could eat anything I wanted to—and I did. These days, though, I teach only five classes, and I must watch what I eat, and the Zumba Diet helps me do that.

SEE LESS OF YOURSELF

How soon will you see results? Let's just say if you follow what I have for you in this book, there could be five to ten pounds less of you within about three weeks, and even more if you stick with it. Easier said than done? Not really, especially if you have carved out time in your schedule for Zumba. You will definitely see your shape change, so do not be afraid to look at yourself in the mirror!

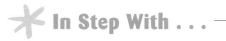 In Step With . . .

Bernice Arias-Sather, Maple Grove, Minneapolis

Four years ago, forty-six-year-old Bernice Arias-Sather received news from her doctor that no one likes to hear: her blood pressure was high, her cholesterol levels were elevated, and she was overweight.

Fortuitously, Bernice saw an infomercial for Zumba, ordered the DVDs, and started Zumba at home.

"You always hear that you should do exercise you enjoy," she recalls. "With Zumba, I really found something that I love and that keeps me motivated."

Bernice has lost fifty pounds since starting Zumba, gotten her health issues under control, and has become a licensed Zumba instructor.

"I love to dance," she said. "I'm not a dancer by trade; it's just in my blood. I'm Hispanic, and in my house I grew up with music and dancing all the time. Zumba has given me a sense that I can do something. I feel more confident in my abilities."

PARK YOUR WORRIES AT THE DOOR

If you are like most people I know, there is a lot going on in your life. You may be working two jobs to make ends meet. You may have a kid who needs encouragement to do better in school. You may be under pressure to make sales quotas at work. You are trying to hold a significant relationship together. Some days are better than others, but I guarantee that you can be having the worst day, and after you have done an hour of Zumba, you will feel so much better.

Many people believe that activities like meditation are a good form of stress relief, and they are. But for me, sitting in the quiet only leads me to start thinking of all those things nagging at the back of my mind. In Zumba, because you are moving to music, you can let yourself go and feel the rhythms of those smooth Latin beats; then it is easy to let go of all your stresses. Dancing has always boosted my confidence and my happiness, and I know it will do the same for you.

So as you prepare for your Zumba workout, please do not think about what is going on in your life. Park your worries at the door and just have a good time.

I hope you are ready to join the party. If so, expect your life to take on a whole new direction before long. Remember what I said at the beginning? Everything is possible.

Chapter 4
FEEL THE MUSIC

Zumba is all about movement. Arms pumping, feet stomping, hips swaying, and, of course, sweat dripping. Now I know you are reading this, saying, "Yeah, that's great, but there is no way my body will ever move in the Zumba way!"

The key to the Zumba fitness program is not flashy choreography; it is the music. Music adds instant energy to your workout. It pulls you in. It makes you want to move. It is very inviting, very sensual. You follow the steps by feeling and moving to the music.

Zumba Fitness music is not the synchronized, synthesized monotonous beat you have heard in many aerobics classes. While that type of music works well for various fitness formats such as step, kickboxing, and so forth, Zumba's uniqueness puts it in a different category. That is why we use the originality, passion, feel, and flow of the song as intended by the music's artist, rather than the syncro-syntho-mono beat. Our music is not simply background music or a way to keep a beat; it is the driving force of Zumba.

The DVD with this book features one hour of energetic, uplifting music. I guarantee that once you hear it, you will just give in to it and start moving your body. Once you are doing that, you are dancing, and you are practicing good health and fitness. Forget about expensive equipment, too. All you need is your body and the willingness to have fun.

 ## In Step With . . .

Suzanne Wells, Northport, New York

Suzanne has been involved in all sorts of creative movement for years. By the time she discovered Zumba, she had already been a group exercise instructor for more than twenty-two years, teaching floor aerobics, step aerobics, group resistance training, yoga, and many specialty exercise classes. "Group fitness provides me with the endorphins I needed, and yoga sustains my spiritual life. However, music always feeds my soul."

When a curious Suzanne walked into her first Zumba class, she understood immediately that this form of dance was much more than a fitness fad. "It allowed me to move organically to music deeply entrenched in culture and let me find my own 'inner rhythm.'"

To Suzanne, Zumba is a unique way to express movement outside of the strict limits of conventional fitness classes and their often strict limits of expression. "In every class I teach and take now, I understand these international rhythms are moving students in their own unique way. I see glowing faces and glistening skin and light in people's eyes. Mostly, their hearts seem lighter. When they go home, I know their day will be better and so will their lives. What could be better than that?"

GETTING TO KNOW LATIN RHYTHMS

The rich variety of Latin music provides an unlimited range of songs and tempos for Zumba. You can use them to create your own workout—and do it right at home.

It is important to learn how to identify the various Latin rhythms, namely the merengue, salsa, cumbia, and reggaeton, so that you can match the steps and the moves to songs. Learning how to identify these rhythms is not something that will occur in a day, a week, or even a month. With time and experience, however, you will get to know these rhythms and be able to differentiate among them. This knowledge will make your Zumba experience even more enjoyable. I will help you get started in this chapter.

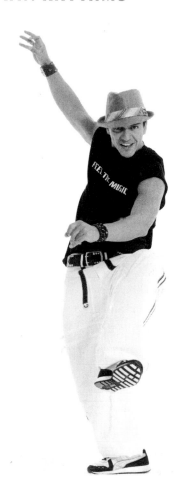

THE FASCINATING HISTORY
OF LATIN RHYTHMS

While teaching Zumba workshops, I explain the history of the dances. I feel very strongly that people need to know where the music comes from, to talk about the path from Africa to Latin America, and the parallel developments in the U.S. Knowledge of dance history makes a difference in how you hear the music, hear the beats, and, ultimately, in how you dance. Everything just sinks in better when you understand the origin of these wonderful dances. So first let's go back in time and discover the rich, fascinating heritage of these dances.

Merengue

The merengue (pronounced *me-RREN-gay*) was born in the Dominican Republic as the music and dance of the lower classes. Because of its close relation with African music and its controversial lyrical content, the dance was spurned by the Dominican upper crust. This changed with the regime of the all-powerful dictator Rafael Leonidas Trujillo. Trujillo, who shared peasant roots with the merengue and loved the dance, forced the rhythm into Dominican high society after he rose to power. In 1930, the merengue became the national dance of the Dominican Republic on his orders. However, Trujillo quickly clamped down on the social commentary prevalent in much of the lyrics.

When you dance a traditional merengue, you keep the part of the body from the waist up very straight, very stiff. This is from the history of the dance. The merengue was first danced during the Haitian occupation of the Dominican Republic from 1822 to 1844. Most men carried guns or rifles at all times, even on the dance floor. With a carbine hanging from your shoulder, it is hard to move your back, so they did not, and today you don't, either. Most merengue action is in the legs and hips.

Why is it called "merengue"? There are several theories. One of the most popular has to do with meringue, the delightful pie and cake topping made of sugar and egg whites. This theory asserts that the name came from an association between the way the meringue is whipped and the way the merengue is danced. The swirling and fast-paced steps by the dancers with the man and the woman's legs crisscrossing remind you of the beating of eggs while preparing the meringue topping.

After attaining great popularity in the Dominican Republic, the infectious merengue spread abroad in the early 1930s by means of radio broadcasts and recorded music. The first areas it reached were places like Puerto Rico, Aruba, Venezuela, and New York City. After conquering those markets, the rhythm's popularity spanned out throughout the rest of the world. By the end of the 1990s, the merengue was monopolizing airplay in most Hispanic Caribbean radio stations and was a favorite at many dance clubs.

Merengue is four-beat dance in which a step is taken for every count. Each merengue beat has the same accent. When you listen to the merengue, it goes 1-2-3-4, with the same accent on all four beats. Diagrammed, the merengue accented beat looks like this:

1	2	3	4	1	2	3	4
same	same	same	same	same	same	same	same

We call beats like this "marching beats," and that is why the basic merengue step is a march. The merengue beat is normally a pulsating up-tempo beat. Dancers add spins, dips, and other fancy moves. Dance-wise, the merengue is so simple that people in dance clubs can get up and dance it without any formal instruction. If you can walk, you can learn the merengue. It is just that easy! You will see just how easy when you play the DVD included with this book.

Salsa

The roots of salsa music and dance can be traced to the early rhythms of Africa as well as southern Spain, although some maintain that the salsa we know today was created in Cuba. Still others say its roots lie in Colombia or Puerto Rico. Salsa was basically a street dance, made popular by Puerto Rican immigrants in New York City in the 1950s and danced in the ghettos. Its steps are a combination of mambo steps with some rumba, some lindy hop, some hustle, and other moves thrown in for flash and style. To me, it is an urban melting pot of many different kinds of Latin steps.

For many years, salsa was considered working-class music, and lower-class expression. Today, the passion for this dance is worldwide: It is danced throughout Europe, South America, Canada, South Africa, Japan, and China, with as many variations as there are people dancing it. Salsa was, and is, multi-cultural, multi-national, and multi-musical.

There are few hard and fast rules about how to perform the dance and plenty of room for individual interpretation and expression. In most styles of salsa, dancers lightly touch or tap the floor with their toes on the first beat. On the second beat, they step back (or front) with the same foot, straightening their knees while transfering their weight and lifting the stationary foot. On the third beat they move their weight back to the center, and on the fourth count, they bring their feet together. The same pattern is then repeated on the other leg.

If you listen to the salsa, it sounds like it has only three beats, but there are actually four beats. The beats are grouped together in such a way that beats 1 through 3 are accented, and the fourth beat is almost silent. It is this arrangement that gives salsa music its distinctive flavor. This sounds complicated, especially if you are new to Latin rhythms, but after you listen to salsa music long enough, you will quickly become accustomed to it, and dancing to its beat will become second nature. Here is what the salsa accents look like when diagrammed:

1	2	3	4	1	2	3	4
hard	medium	medium	soft	hard	medium	medium	soft

You will notice that beat 1 is accented the most strongly. This is because it is the introductory beat of the rhythm. Salsa is the fastest tempo of the four basic rhythms in Zumba, as you will discover on the companion DVD.

While the basic step is simple, there are many ways to spice it up. (After all, the word *salsa* literally means "sauce," a spicy mixture that gives flavor.) You can focus on moving your hips in the same direction as your step, for example. This gives you the desired sensual look of the dance.

On the dance floor and in clubs, salsa is a partner dance. Traditionally, the man does the leading. During the dance, partners rarely speak to each other, but use eye contact and subtle hand and body signals to communicate a change in step—much like a Zumba instructor does when leading a class.

I love salsa. To me, it is more than a dance. It is life, the motion of intense rhythm, being in the beat and on top of the world.

Reggaeton

Reggaeton is actually a form of dance music that originated in Panama and Puerto Rico. Featuring a driving drum-machine track, it was, and still is, the undisputed favorite of urban kids. Lyrically, reggaeton blends rapping and singing, hip-hop, and funk. Its infectious rhythm is known for making people want to dance.

Reggaeton is said first to have arrived in Latin America with Jamaican laborers who came to help build the Panama Canal in the early twentieth century. By the early 1980s, the music could be heard across much of Latin America, though it was considered underground. Puerto Rican musicians translated the Jamaican version into Spanish, and when these lyrics were fused with Panamanian-style beats, reggaeton was born. A mix of hip-hop, merengue, rap, and other Caribbean styles, the genre became hugely popular in Puerto Rico by the mid-1990s. Just as rap has been a symbol for urban youth in North America, reggaeton became, and remains, a defining symbol of urban youth in Latin America, specifically Puerto Rico.

Reggaeton percolated for years in the streets and clubs of Puerto Rico before making its way to the United States. Its infectious, driving rhythms and the sexy bump-and-grind dancing that it inspires made it a favorite in clubs, particularly in such cities as New York and Miami. What really made it explode in these cities was so much demand in the Latin community.

The reggaeton definitely has four beats, but they are usually grouped together as two sets of four, or a total of eight beats. The first beat is a very strong one:

1	2	3	4	5	6	7	8
hard	soft	medium	medium	**hard**	soft	medium	medium

The reggaeton is a lively, pounding beat. When dancing to reggaeton, you use foot shuffles, hip movements, slides, and other hip-hop moves. Reggaeton happens to be one of my favorite rhythms. It loosens the hips and really works the entire body. Its high-intensity dance movements and urban sounds definitely work up a sweat. Reggaeton dance steps are high-intensity cardio moves.

Cumbia

At the heart of my upbringing was the cumbia (pronounced *KUM-bee-yah*), a hypnotic danceable rhythm that originated in the 1800s as part of the Spanish slave trade in Colombian coastal areas. Historically, it was a courtship ritual between African men and Indian women at a time when the two communities were intermarrying in Colombia.

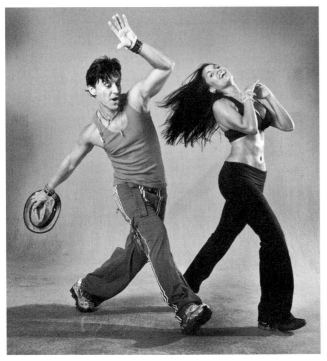

Symbolic of a man trying to win a woman's heart, the ritual was rhythmically performed by men-and-women couples. The women playfully waved with their long skirts and held a candle, while the men danced behind them. The men kept one hand behind their backs, and held their hats in the other, putting them on and taking them off and waving them. Men also carried a red bandana that they wrapped around their necks, waved in circles in the air, or hand-held with their partners. Until the mid-twentieth century, cumbia was practiced only by the lower classes.

ZUMBA FITNESS TIP:
"Drum" Health and Fitness into Your Life

Many Zumba classes around the world incorporate live drumming as part of the music. Drumming can be a powerful tool when combined with exercise. It enhances many of the physical and emotional effects of exercise, including intensity of effort, stress reduction, and the release of endorphins. In fact, many Zumba participants find they get "charged up" by the sound of drumming. This effect increases their energy and motivation even more while working out.

If you think about it, our bodies are rhythmic: our blood flows, our heart beats, and our lungs breathe in patterns. So it is no wonder our bodies innately respond to the rhythms of drumming. If you feel out of sync or cannot keep up with the pressures of your busy lifestyle, consider listening to some drum music.

Interestingly, drumming is being used effectively in the treatment of many conditions, such as diabetes, asthma, cancer, cardiovascular and chronic lung disease, post-traumatic stress disorder, and depression. It is also showing promise with diseases and disorders like Alzheimer's, multiple sclerosis, paralysis, Parkinson's, and multiple personality disorder.

How does drumming affect these disorders? Researchers have found that when people with irregular or weak brain rhythms, such as individuals with Alzheimer's disease, listened to music with strong rhythms, their brain waves became more organized, pronounced, and higher in frequency. While the research is still in its infancy, it suggests that music, and drumming in particular, may have a healing effect on the brain.

The dance traditionally was, and in the case of many folkloric groups, still is, danced barefoot. One story has it that the dance originated with slaves who were chained together and, of necessity, were forced to drag one leg as they cut sugar cane to the beat of drums. This is why today we drag our feet as part of the cumbia dance steps.

The movement imparts a very soft feeling, with a step that slows the pace and allows you to dip back and forth on the balls of your feet and wave your arms up and down like palms swaying to an offshore breeze. There is a lot of hip movement, too. Though cumbia is typically a partner dance, it can be done in large groups, and this has made it very popular.

Cumbia sounds much like salsa with its four equally accented beats. There is a soft beat in between each accented beat, however. It feels like: 1 *and* 2 *and* 3 *and* 4. Visually, the cumbia beat looks like this:

1	and	2	and	3	and	4
hard	soft	**hard**	soft	**hard**	soft	**hard**

The "and" beat is almost like a hiccup between the hard beats. Also, the cumbia beat is slower than the other Latin rhythms. In the basic cumbia step, your front foot is the hard, accented beat, and your back foot is the "and." The lilting cumbia is a good rhythm for slowing the pace in a Zumba workout.

I dance the cumbia all the time when I have the opportunity. It is very emotional for me. It is my culture. It is something I have known all my life.

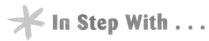 ## In Step With . . .

Karen Blanchard, Portland, Maine

After years of broken New Year's resolutions to lose weight, Karen Blanchard dropped ten dress sizes and shed sixty pounds off her five-foot-four-inch frame after discovering Zumba on an infomercial and doing it on a regular basis.

"Exercise is in and of itself is such a hard thing for a lot of women and men," Karen said. "When you find something you really love to do, it's wonderful."

A licensed Zumba instructor, Karen loves Zumba so much that she opened her own studio and generated a huge clientele.

"I love being able to offer a workout for people discouraged by the grind of traditional aerobics classes."

Another way to identify a rhythm is by its instruments. Here is a look at the instruments normally played in each type of Latin rhythm:

RHYTHM	INSTRUMENTS
Merengue	*Tambora* (a double-headed drum played with one stick and the hand), *Congo drums*, *trumpets*, and *guiro* (percussion instrument made of a hollow gourd, played by scraping with a stick or rod)
Salsa	*Timbales* (metal drums), *Congo drums*, *clave* (a percussion instrument consisting of two small wooden sticks that are hit together to produce a high-pitched sound), *trumpet*, and *trombone*
Cumbia	*Guiro, accordion*, and *tambora*
Reggaeton	*Bass drum*

We will learn the basic Zumba steps in the next chapter, and you will discover how simple they are. But here is what I want you to remember: All Zumba moves come alive when you relax, listen carefully to the rhythm, feel it, enjoy it, and, of course, have fun!

Chapter 5
ZUMBA: STEP BY STEP

Okay, have you always wanted to learn salsa or merengue? Here is your chance to fulfill a dream and get in shape at the same time.

In this chapter I am going to demonstrate how to do the four basic steps of Zumba: salsa, merengue, cumbia, and reggaeton. Each step is broken down into its basic components and described in the text. Also, each step is clearly demonstrated in photographs that accompany the text—and in the companion DVD. You can master all these steps by studying this chapter and watching the DVD. It is a great tool for learning the rhythms.

Ultimately, these steps form the building blocks of the Zumba workouts, along with my sculpt-and-tone moves, which I introduce in Chapter 6. You will first learn the steps here and the sculpt-and-tone moves next. Then we will put everything together in Chapter 7, with the Zumba workouts.

But you are probably wondering: Can I learn and master the Zumba dance steps and rhythms from a book? You bet you can! In fact, a book like this is one of the best ways to learn to dance because the directions are spelled out for you, the moves are illustrated and shown on the DVD, and you can absorb the information and practice the steps at your own pace. Not only that, you can study the photographs and imprint the images in your mind for easy recall when you get ready to do Zumba.

I suggest that you work on one or two steps a day to build your confidence and competence. Then move on to another one or two steps, and so on, until you can practically do Zumba in your sleep. As you practice in this manner, you will be on your way to getting a shapely, sexy body, since the different dance steps give different benefits. For instance, salsa and reggaeton emphasize a cardiovascular workout, so overall fat-burning is the result. On the other hand, certain aspects of merengue and cumbia focus more on strengthening specific body parts—hips, thighs, legs, and stomach muscles—as well as fostering greater endurance.

LET'S DANCE!

What you are about to experience, learn, and practice are some of my best booty-shaking, hip-swaying moves. Spiced with lively beats, these steps are a snap. I do recommend that you study the DVD, too. It is like having your own personal Zumba instructor by your side.

You can learn Zumba right in your living room or getting down as you wash dishes. No special equipment is needed other than inspiring, motivating music that you can dance passionately to and let yourself go. If you are uninhibited, trust me, you will burn plenty of calories. And if you are at home, you are bound to be less inhibited! Remember, feel the music, too. When you are inspired by music, you will want to move. Music is a motion, and dancing allows you to interpret music through your body.

Are you ready? Let's go!

THE FOUR BASIC STEPS

You will be surprised by how easy these steps are to learn. I will outline how to perform each step, then I will teach you some variations. Each basic step has the following variations:

* Arm variations to help work your upper body.

* Fitness (body toning) variations like lunges or squats to help you strengthen and tone specific body parts.

* Directional variations (side to side, a circle, or stepping up and back), in order to add some extra flair to the step.

What I would like you to do is read through the rest of this chapter carefully to get familiar with the steps and their variations. Look closely at the photographs. Then slowly walk through each step and variation several times before moving on to the next one. Develop a real familiarity with the moves so they begin to feel like second nature.

Make sure you have plenty of space to practice. Any room of the house is fine; just make sure it is open, with all the furniture pushed back and out of the way. If you're ready, I'm ready. Let's get started.

THE MERENGUE

The Merengue March

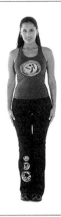

Start: Begin the march with your feet together and your arms at your sides.

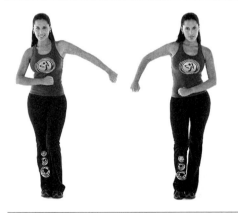

Action: Start marching right and left. Let your hips naturally sway in time with your foot movements. To engage your hips, allow your knees to turn inward a bit. If your hips do not move well, that's okay; just keep marching. Your arms should move naturally, the right arm going up as the left knee goes down, and the left arm going up as the right knee goes down.

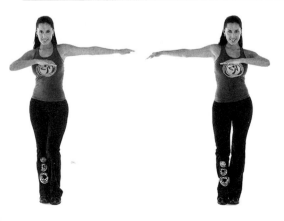

Arm Variation 1: Lift your arms straight out to your sides at about shoulder level.

Bend your right elbow and bring your right hand to chest level; straighten your arm back out. Bend your left elbow and bring your left hand to chest level; straighten your arm back out. Bend and straighten your arms like this in an alternating fashion as you march. This arm variation resembles a waving motion.

Arm Variation 2: Push your arms up toward the ceiling.

Then bring them back down to chest level.

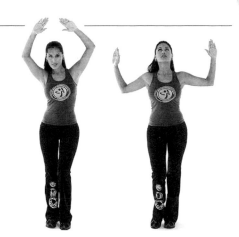

Next, bring your arms down to the front of your chest.

Then extend your arms out to your sides. Repeat this sequence as you march in time to the music.

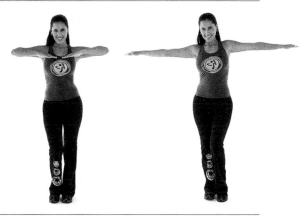

Directional Variation: Take your march forward 4 steps and back 4 steps. You can also go around in a circle: March to your right 4 steps forward and 4 steps back, then return to the center. March to the back, 4 steps forward and 4 steps back, then return to center. March to the left for 4 steps forward and 4 steps back, then return to the center.

Fitness Variation: Open your legs slightly wider than shoulder-distance apart as you march, still swaying your hips from side to side. Let your arms move naturally, or try one of the arm variations. This move engages your core. You should also feel it in your quads.

The Side-to-Side Merengue

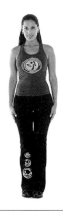 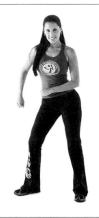

Start: Begin this step with your feet together, and arms held naturally at your sides.

Action: Next, step out to your right side on your right foot. Swing your hips as you step out.

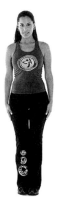 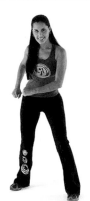

Then return to the center starting position.

Step out to your left side on your left foot. Swing your hips as you step out.

Then return to the center starting position.

Alternate in this fashion, swinging your hips. Let your arms move naturally, or feel free to add one of the arm variations illustrated earlier.

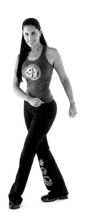 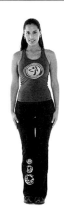

Directional Variation: With your left leg, step over to your right, crossing over your right leg.

Return to the center starting position.

With your right leg, step over to your left, crossing over your left leg.

Alternate in this fashion, swinging your hips. Let your arms move naturally, or feel free to add one of the arm variations illustrated earlier.

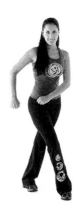

Fitness Variation (Lunge): Step out to your right side, then lunge on your right leg. Return to the center starting position. Step out to your left side, then lunge on your left leg. Return to the center starting position. Alternate in this fashion.

Fitness Variation (Squat): Step out to your right side, then squat by bending both knees. Place your hands on your thighs as you squat. Squeeze your buttocks muscles. Return to the center starting position. Step out to your left side, then squat on your left leg, keeping your hands on your thighs. Return to the center starting position. Alternate in this fashion.

The Beto Shuffle

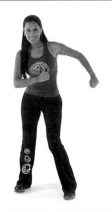

Start: This is my signature merengue step for Zumba. Like most Zumba steps, it uses every muscle of your body and gives you a great full-body workout.

Begin with your feet shoulder-distance apart, knees slightly bent, and your arms ready to move, as shown. During this move, your feet stay fairly planted on the floor. You merely pivot on the balls of your feet as you turn from side to side.

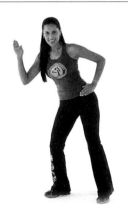

Action: Angle one forearm up, and angle the other forearm down, as pictured. Your feet will follow your arms in small "shuffling" side-to-side steps. Keep your left foot planted and bend your left knee slightly as you turn your body to the right. Shuffle twice on your right foot. Simultaneously angle your right forearm up and your left hand on your hip, as shown.

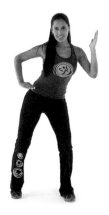

Then twist your body to the other side.

Do the same move in the opposite direction, but shuffle once on your left foot. The sequence of Beto Shuffle is typically: right, right, left, right; then left, left, right, left.

Directional Variation: Do the same move, but turn in a circle, first to the right, then to the left.

Fitness Variation: Bend your knees into a near-squat position as you perform the shuffle. This variation works your thighs.

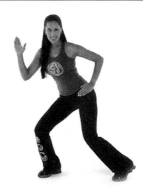

SALSA

The Cuban Step

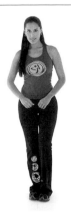 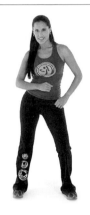

Start: Stand with your feet together, with your arms at your waist.

Action: Step out to the left, shifting your weight to your left leg.

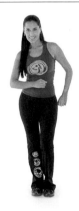 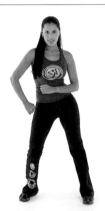

Return to the starting position.

Step out to the right, shifting your weight to your right leg.

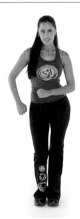

Return to the starting position.

Repeat this sequence, letting your arms move naturally. Try to add a little more hip swaying as you move.

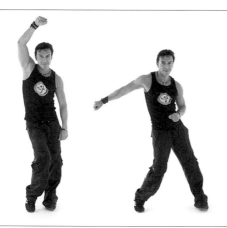

Arm Variation 1: Extend your right arm to the ceiling.

Bring it down, across your chest. Then sweep it out to your side at shoulder level. Imagine you are drawing an L in the air with your arm. Repeat with your left arm. Alternate, one arm at a time.

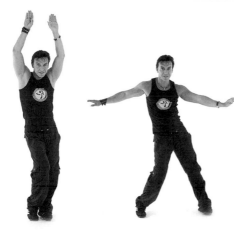

Arm Variation 2: This move is similar to Arm Variation 1, except that you will move both arms simultaneously. Extend both arms to the ceiling.

Bring them down, across your chest. Then sweep both arms out to your sides at shoulder level. Imagine you are drawing L's in the air with your arms.

Fitness Variation: This variation involves doing a squat and works your thighs and glutes. Begin with your feet together.

Step out to the right.

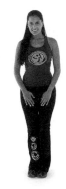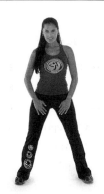

Squat so that your thighs are parallel to the floor, as shown.

Return to the starting position. Repeat, stepping out to the left.

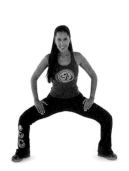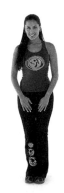

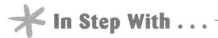

✳ In Step With . . .

Elizabeth Gigler, Palos Hills, Illinois

Elizabeth Gigler began a career in the fitness industry about twenty years ago as an aerobics instructor. Back then, she was a young single mother who taught aerobics part-time to get in shape and make some extra money. Amazingly, she taught a class the day before she gave birth to her daughter. "I remember telling the ladies at the gym that my daughter was already so used to the music that she was going to come into the world doing aerobics," she says.

Elizabeth continued to teach part-time and got involved in all of the fitness trends, from step aerobics to kickboxing to yoga. "It wasn't until I was in my thirties that I started to slow down. I thought it was just getting older. Turns out I had a medical condition that ultimately ended with me having a hysterectomy. Those years right before and right after were the worst. I stopped working out completely."

Elizabeth began putting on weight and was later diagnosed with rheumatoid arthritis. Sitting around was just making life worse, and Elizabeth knew she had to do something. Fortunately, the spa where she had been employed was open to letting her come back to teach. She heard the manager mention that the spa wanted to add Zumba to the schedule.

"I had never heard of Zumba, but thought it sounded like opportunity knocking. I looked up Zumba online and knew I had to give it a try," she says. "I was a little concerned about all the weight I had gained, but it looked like so much fun. I signed up for the next instructor training and told my manager I would be ready to teach at the start of the new year.

"Taking that workshop inspired me to really put my workouts into high gear. I had about a month before my first class, so I practiced every night after I came home from my desk job. My now teenage daughter would see me practicing, but rather than laugh at her old mom, she would stand alongside me and help me practice."

When the New Year came, the gym launched a big Zumba party to get everyone excited. "The members loved it as much as I did."

A year later, Elizabeth found herself fifty pounds lighter. Remember the daughter she predicted would come into the world doing aerobics? The prediction came true in a way: Elizabeth's daughter is now a licensed Zumba instructor.

"It is so much fun having two Zumba instructors in the family," Elizabeth says. "The members really enjoy having us both up there. Zumba not only changed me physically, it gave me something fun to share with my daughter."

The Salsa Back Step

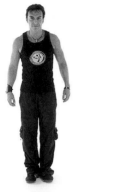 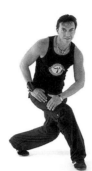

Start: Begin with your feet together, with your arms at your sides.

Action: Step back with your left foot, turning your shoulders and twisting your body slightly to the left and tapping your left foot to the back.

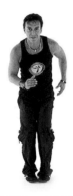 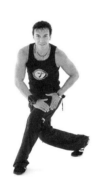

Return to center.

Repeat to the right side. Step back with your right foot, turning your shoulders and twisting your body slightly to the right and tapping your right foot to the back. Return to center.

Your arms should follow your legs. For example, when your left leg goes back, your left arm goes back.

Arm Variation: As you twist back, let your arms swing down to your sides. Then as you twist forward, extend your arms upward. Extending your arms upward helps raise your heart rate.

Fitness Variation: Facing forward, lift your right knee; then lower your right leg to the back. Lift your left knee; then lower your left leg to the back. Continue alternating in this fashion for extra emphasis on the thighs.

The Basic Salsa

Start: Begin with your feet together and arms at your sides.

Action: Step forward on your left foot.

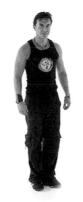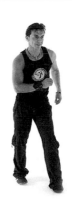

Then bring your right foot to meet it and close your feet.

Next, step forward on your right foot.

Then bring your left foot to meet it and close your feet.

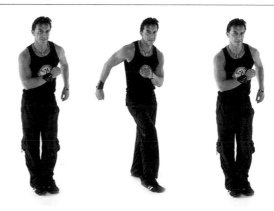

Step back on your left foot.

Then bring your right foot to meet it and close your feet.

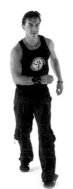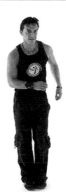

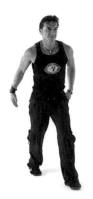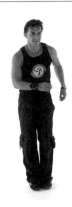

Next, step back on your right foot.

Then bring your left foot to meet it and close your feet. Repeat this sequence.

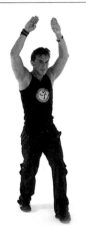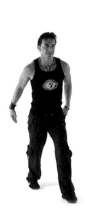

Arm Variation: As you step forward, extend your arms overhead. As you step backward, swing your arms down and back. Combine this move naturally with the steps, and you will really work your body.

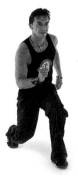

Fitness Variation: Each time you step forward, lunge on your lead leg.

CUMBIA

The Basic Cumbia

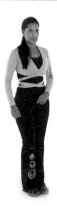

Start: Turn your body slightly to the side, as shown. Stand with your feet together. Distribute your weight evenly on both feet.

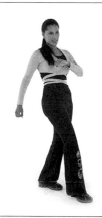 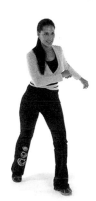

Action: Start with your right leg. Swing your right leg forward, keeping your left foot stationary. Tap your right foot toward the front. Swing your left arm forward with it, and let your right arm swing toward the back.

Next, swing your right foot to the back and tap it toward the back. Keep your weight on your left leg through the sequence.

Let your hips follow the movement of your leg. Repeat this forward-back sequence. Really try to engage your hips and your core. You can twist slightly at the waist as you move, and this really works your oblique muscles at the sides of your waist.

Turn to the opposite side, and repeat the sequence with your left leg, swinging your arms in the process.

Note: With the cumbia, I do not employ arm variations as much as I add fitness and directional variations.

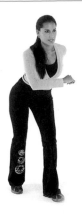

Fitness Variation: Lean forward slightly. As you bring your leg back, try to take it back as far as you can. This variation engages your quads and your abs.

The Sugar Cane

Start: Begin with your feet together. Place your right hand on your hip and extend your left arm up, as shown.

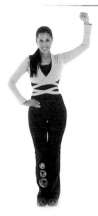

Action: With your left leg, step forward, and step back to center.

Switch sides and do the move with your right leg. As you move your right leg through this pattern, your left leg stays in place, although you pivot on the ball of your left foot.

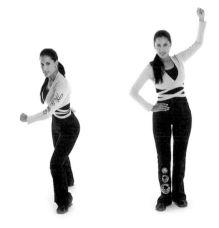

Arm Variation: As you take the forward step, make a downward chopping movement with your free hand (the other hand remains on your hip). As you step center and back, swing your free arm up behind you. This arm variation mimics the motion of cutting down sugar cane in the fields.

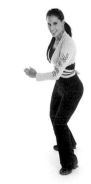

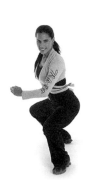 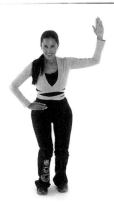

Fitness Variation (Squat): As you step forward, bend both knees and go into a squat.

Then step to the center, and squat. The step sequence is as follows: squat forward, squat center, step back, and step center.

The Sleepy Leg

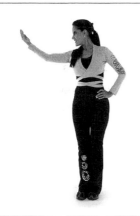

Start: Begin with your feet together. Place your left hand on your left hip, with the right arm outstretched.

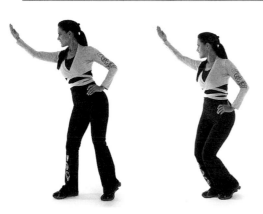

Action: Step to your right side with your right foot.

Then drag your left foot to meet your right foot.

Repeat this move 4 times, then switch sides. Twist at the waist for a bit of flair as you move.

Arm Variation: Extend both arms out to shoulder level to engage the upper body.

Directional Variation: Turn in a circle as you step forward, step forward, step center, step back, and step center.

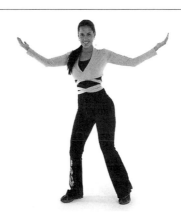

REGGAETON

The Reggaeton Basic

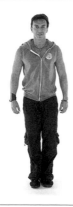

Start: Begin with your feet together and your arms at your sides. This is a simple step-touch movement.

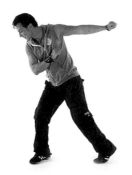 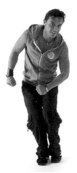

Action: Step out to the right side with your right foot.

Then bring your left foot to touch it.

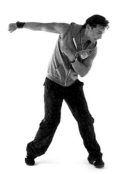 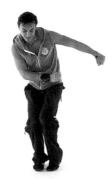

Step out to the left side with your left foot.

Then bring your right foot to touch it.

Step-touch, step-touch, back and forth, back and forth. To add reggaeton flair, swing your arms in the opposite direction from your body.

For a different pattern, you can do a single step-touch, followed by a double step-touch. In a double, you simply perform two step-touches in a row in the same direction.

Directional Variation: Turn to the right, do a double step-touch, followed by a single step-touch. Turn to the back and repeat. Turn to the side and repeat. Turn to the front and repeat the move to all four walls.

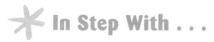

✳ In Step With . . .

Cindy Samudio, Houston, Texas

Cindy Samudio, a forty-seven-year-old mother of two, had struggled to lose weight after the birth of her second child, but it just wasn't coming off.

"I can honestly say that I wasn't putting a lot of intensity into my workouts. I was just going through the motions," she said. "I was even on one of those meal plans where you weigh in and buy your food for the week. I think I actually gained a pound or two on that program."

In December 2004, a frustrated Cindy decided to try something different: yoga. She fell in love with it and could feel her body strengthening and toning up, though her weight had not dropped much.

Cindy's yoga instructor asked her if she had ever considered teaching yoga, since her form and technique were so good. Inspired, Cindy became a yoga instructor.

There was only one problem: her weight. "I've got to lose this weight now that I'm teaching in front of all these people," Cindy told herself. She began making more balanced meals with more vegetables and fruit, and a few more pounds came off.

About three months into her career as a yoga instructor, Cindy was asked to be a Zumba instructor. She was game, and so she practiced at home with Zumba Fitness DVDs prior to teaching classes. Once she started teaching Zumba classes three times a week, the rest of her weight just seemed to melt right off. In fact, Cindy lost twenty-five pounds in just two months. Ultimately, she dropped from 150 pounds to 115 pounds, and went from a dress size of 11½ to a size 4.

"This is my life now," she said. "I wouldn't trade it for anything. I absolutely love what I do. It's not about trying to be a 'Skinny Minnie.' It's about my health and improving my quality of life. We're only given this one body, and it's up to us to care for it as best we can."

The Reggaeton Stomp

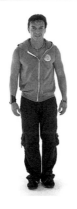

Start: Begin with your feet together and your arms at your sides.

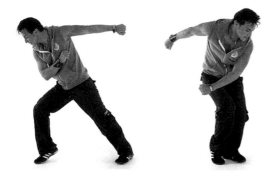

Action: Step sideways on your right leg—and stomp your right foot.

As you stomp, your hip moves in the direction of your foot. Return to center.

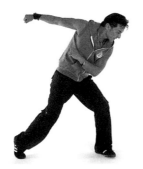

Repeat with your left leg. Lean your upper body forward slightly, keeping your abs engaged. Add some forward shoulder rolls for a little attitude. This is a fun, fun move!

For a different pattern, you can step forward on your right leg—and stomp your right foot twice (a double stomp). Follow this with a single stomp on the same leg. Repeat with your left leg.

Directional Variation: Turn to the right, do a double stomp followed by a single stomp. Turn to the back, do a double stomp followed by a single stomp. Turn to the side, do a double stomp followed by a single stomp. Turn to the front, do a double stomp followed by a single stomp.

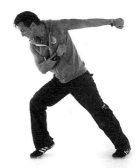

Fitness Variation: When you stomp, lunge forward slightly to work your thighs.

ZUMBA FITNESS TIP:

Visualize the Moves

Here is something you might want to try to improve the execution of the steps: visualization. This is the re-creation of an image or experience in your mind. Start by seeing in your mind's eye the specific movements of each dance step. As an example, go through all the basic components of the merengue in your head, including the arm variations. When your brain imagines your body going through the moves, it sends small impulses via your nervous system to the actual muscles used to perform this step. Visualization establishes a nerve pathway between your brain and the muscles associated with that action. So when you physically practice a movement, your brain will recall how it has stored the directions for that movement and will send the correct signals directly to the muscles.

The Reggaeton Bounce

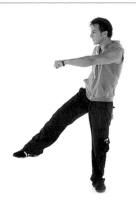

Start: Begin with your feet wider than hip width. Turn your body to the right, lifting your right knee and reaching your left arm out.

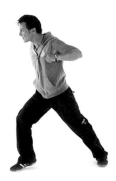

Action: Step out onto your right foot as you pump your left arm back, pulling your chest through and traveling to the right. Repeat this move on the other side.

All of the above steps can be easily translated into constant activity—in other words, a routine set to music. And that's what you will learn to do in Chapter 7: follow a Zumba routine based on the moves you have been learning. Before we get to that, I want to show you some body-toning exercises that can be worked into your routine, too.

Chapter 6

ZUMBA SCULPT, TONE, AND STRETCH

Here is where you can spice up your Zumba routine a little more—with my special sculpt, tone, and stretch moves. Virtually everyone longs for a toned, in-shape body, yet many people spin their wheels without making significant long-term progress. As a fitness instructor, I hear men and women complain time and again about their "trouble zones"—those sagging, wiggly parts that seem resistant to diet or exercise. But I have also seen what works to firm and tighten them: spot-toning, which is what my Zumba sculpt, tone, and stretch exercises do for you, while infusing the irresistible element of fun into the workout.

Essentially, these exercises initiate the body-sculpting process by refining the muscles developed through cardio. You will learn how to spot-tone with truly amazing results, from flatter abs to a tighter butt to sleeker thighs to a firmer body overall. Your mind will also reap benefits, including lowered stress and a greater sense of body awareness and confidence. Twenty minutes, two to three times a week: that's all it takes to firm your butt, abs, thighs, and other jiggly body parts you thought were impossible to tighten. My moves reshape these tough-to-tone areas by isolating one or two muscles at a time and making them work hard without much help from other muscles. The result: You lose inches and recontour the problem spots. Pretty good for such a time-efficient routine. And while you will find some old favorites here, you will also spot fresh takes on familiar moves.

These moves are especially popular if you do not want to venture into the weight room, since they can be easily done at home. Many people are uncomfortable with, intimidated by, or unsure of how to use exercise machines, or they fear bulking up. Don't worry; you will not bulk up, I promise. Using lighter hand weights, as well as your body's own weight, makes this less likely.

ZUMBA FITNESS TIP:

Toning Techniques

* Challenge your muscles with resistance, either with my toning sticks or light dumbbells. These will let you consistently perform exercises with excellent form.

* Keep up your Zumba cardio work. It not only uses large muscle groups rhythmically, it also makes your heart pump harder to burn calories and oxygen.

* Do not use momentum (swinging your arms or rocking your body) to help you lift the weights or carry you through reps. Resist on every move—and really feel it.

* Focus on quality, not quantity. One hundred reps are useless if they are done incorrectly.

Best of all, you can perform these moves to motivating, uplifting Zumba Fitness music. You know yourself that if exercise is just repetitive exercise, it can become boring. But when done to the accompaniment of music, you enjoy it more, and you stay in the groove. It is easier to concentrate on the natural feel of the exercises, and the parts of your body that are being used. This focus on isolating muscle groups can have a meditative quality as well, especially with my Zumba stretches. All in all, concentrating on working individual parts of the body while moving to music creates a new kind of liaison between body and brain that you may never have sensed before. With this kind of focus, you will get better results.

With many of these moves, you can use my special Zumba "toning sticks" or any type of light (two-to-three-pound) dumbbells in your workout. These supply external resistance so that you build lean muscle and your body becomes even more efficient at burning fat. These innovative moves work your muscles in an integrated way to boost flexibility and strength as well as body awareness. I believe one of the keys to getting measurable results is thinking about what you are doing. Try to engage your mind before you engage your muscles. Do each move slowly and fluidly, inhaling and exhaling through your nose.

One more point: You will see that some of these moves include some basic Zumba steps, thus working your upper and lower body at the same time. With this sort of combination work, you can increase your heart rate, burn more calories and fat, plus sculpt your body into a fit, firm, just-plain-amazing body.

ZUMBA AB WORK

Because the abdominals are the centerpiece of your body, a flat stomach and small waist will give you a taller, leaner appearance. Unfortunately, most people never reach these goals. But with these moves you will. They help you sculpt and define your entire torso, all the way down to your deepest abdominal layer. By contracting and strengthening all your abdominal muscles at once, you will get a flatter belly and make a "spare tire" less likely.

Booty Circle

Here is an ab-sculpting move adapted from the ancient art of belly dancing. Belly dancing started in the Middle East and now combines influences from Egypt, Turkey, Greece, Lebanon, and Morocco. It works the whole body but is particularly good for the waist. It strengthens the abs and increases flexibility in the lower back and hip joints. This move is basically a hip-circling motion. I have broken it down into four easy motions you can slowly connect at your own pace.

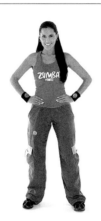 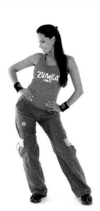

Start: Begin in a standing position. Open your legs about shoulder-distance apart. Place your hands on your hips.

Action: With your feet stable on the floor, lift your right hip up to your right side.

Next, tilt your hips to the back.

Then lift your left hip to your left side.

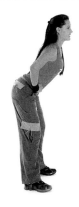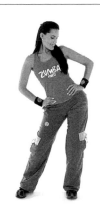

Finally, tilt your hips to the front while contracting your abs with a crunch.

Basically, you are making a circle with your hips: right side, back, left side, front with a crunch. Do not be afraid to stick out your booty!

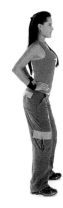

Reggaeton Crunch

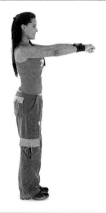

Start: Begin with your legs together. Raise your arms in front of your chest and bend your elbows. Hold your arms in front of your chest, with your forearms and the palms of your hands facing the floor.

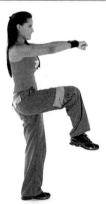

Action: Keeping your left foot stable, lift your right knee up toward your belly button into a knee raise. Contract your abs.

Lower your right leg but do not let it touch the floor. Lift your right knee up again and contract your abs. Repeat this move 4 times with the right leg. Switch legs and do the move 4 times with the left leg.

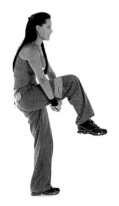

Spice It Up: Lift your knee to your belly button. Bring your arms down and under your knee to meet. Contract your abs.

Tip: Try the Reggaeton Crunch at a faster tempo. Always concentrate on contracting your abs.

Zumba Standing Twist

Start: Stand with your feet a little wider than shoulder-distance apart and keep your knees slightly bent. Place your hands on your hips. Keep your hips stationary to isolate your core.

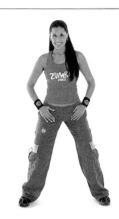

Action: Now twist your upper body from the torso, while reaching across your chest toward the right with your left arm.

Stretch the torso to the right as far as possible.

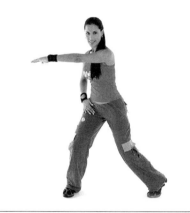

Return to the starting position.

Repeat the move toward the left side.

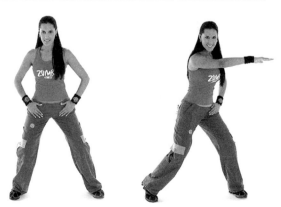

Urban Core Twist

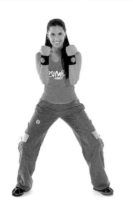

Start: Stand with your legs slightly wider than shoulder-distance apart. Bend your knees slightly. Bring your arms up in front of your chest and bend your elbows. Your upper arms should be nearly parallel to the floor. Hold your fists at about head-height. Keep your hips stationary to isolate your core.

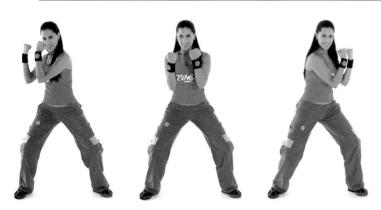

Action: Twist from side to side at the waist in the sequence shown.

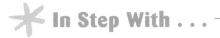 **In Step With . . .**

Kirstyn Niebbia, Warsaw, Indiana

Hitting an all-time-high weight of 240 pounds in 2007 was a moment of truth for Kirstyn Niebbia. She had just given birth to her fifth child, and after a long recovery from a C-section delivery, Kirstyn decided that it was time for a change.

"A friend gave me her Zumba Fitness DVDs. She felt she was not coordinated enough to do them. I laughed, because she is a Latina!"

Kirstyn began following the DVDs every day, in addition to cleaning up her diet. Out went the processed foods that had been causing her weight gain. A year later, she was fifty pounds lighter.

She continued to follow the DVDs daily and began to jog on a treadmill. "For the first time in ten years, I had a waist, and my abs were feeling tight under my still-overweight tummy. I had come this far, and I was not giving up!"

Several months into 2008, Kirstyn weighed "an amazing 160"—less than when she got married, less than when she was fifteen years old.

Then she hit a plateau and the pounds stopped coming off. "I tried everything to shake it up and get off that plateau, but the needle on my scale wouldn't budge."

Kirstyn's stalemate was broken after she became a licensed Zumba instructor. The extra work involved in choreographing and practicing her routines apparently burned up extra calories and revived her metabolism. Kirstyn got on the scale the morning of her first class and was happy to see that, finally, she had dropped more weight—five pounds to be exact. "All I needed to kick my plateau was a little more Zumba!"

ZUMBA ARM WORK

Stop hiding behind long sleeves! Sculpt beautiful arms that you will be proud to bare—and do it without lifting heavier weights, and without doing the same old boring biceps curls. This sequence of moves works your biceps, the arm muscles that come to mind when someone asks you to "flex your muscles." Yes, biceps are for showing off. Curvaceous, toned biceps muscles are sexy and very attractive. Plus, it means you have strong arms. These exercises stabilize your torso and upper arms, forcing you to isolate your biceps so you get strong (yet attractive-looking) arms in record time.

Zumba Curls

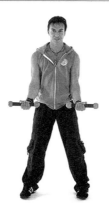

Start: Begin in a standing position, with your legs about shoulder-distance apart. Grasp your toning sticks or light dumbbells (about two to three pounds each) in each hand and let your arms hang straight down at your sides. Flex your knees slightly, as shown.

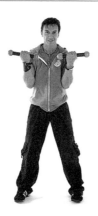

Action: Bend your arms to curl the weights up toward your shoulders. Keep your upper arms close to the sides of your body. Squeeze your biceps in both arms at the top of the movement.

Lower the weights to the starting position.
Repeat the move for a series of repetitions.

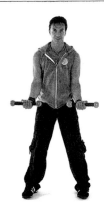

Spice It Up: Next, I want you to do an alternating form of this move. Bend your right arm to curl the weight up to your right shoulder. As you complete the upward movement on the right, begin to curl the left dumbbell up until it reaches your left shoulder, while lowering the right weight. Continue alternating the curl in this fashion for a series of repetitions.

Zumba Triceps Press

This sequence of moves works the triceps muscle at the back of your upper arm. Soft, flabby triceps can greatly detract from your appearance in sleeveless outfits, so let's start working!

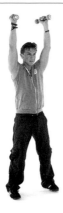

Start: Begin in a standing position, with your legs about shoulder-distance apart. Grasp your toning sticks or light dumbbells in both hands between your crossed thumbs and fingers, behind your head. Flex your knees slightly.

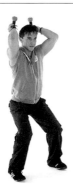

Action: Bend your elbows and lower the weight until it touches your upper back, as shown. At the same time, squat down so that your thighs are just parallel to the floor.

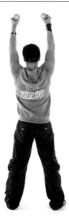

As you straighten your legs, extend your arms straight up, keeping your biceps as close to the side of your head as possible.

ZUMBA SHOULDER AND BACK WORK

For a gorgeous upper body, do exercises that sculpt your back and shoulders and train you to stand tall. The beauty of a toned back and shoulders is lost if you slouch, so I have developed a sequence of moves that does two things at once. First, it helps strengthen and tone your major upper-back and shoulder muscles to create that sexy, sculpted look. Second, the moves are designed to build endurance.

Developing your shoulders and back also gives symmetry to your physique and helps you appear to have a slimmer waist. Strong, toned shoulders correct posture, too, for a look of confidence, grace, and energy. The following moves are an effective way to better endow your shoulder line. Incorporated into your overall Zumba routine, they promise to sculpt your shoulders and upper body into better shape in only a few short weeks.

Zumba Overhead Press

Start: Begin in a standing position, with your legs about shoulder-distance apart. Grasp your toning sticks or light dumbbells in each hand. Hold them up out at your sides, at about shoulder-height, with your palms facing forward and elbows bent, as shown.

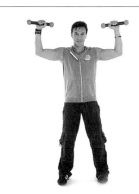

Action: Press the weights upward to an overhead position. Fully extend your elbows at the top of the movement.

Lower the weights to the shoulder-level position.

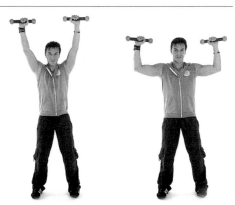

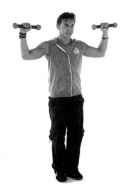

Spice It Up: Begin in a standing position, with your legs about shoulder-distance apart. Grasp your toning sticks or light dumbbells in each hand. Hold them up out at your sides, at about shoulder-height, with your palms facing forward and elbows bent, as shown.

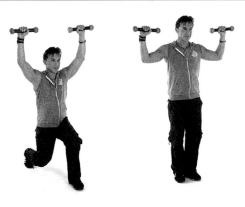

Lunge forward while pressing upward.

Return to the starting position and repeat on the opposite leg.

Zumba Lateral Raise with Squat

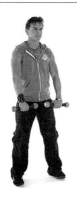

Start: Begin in a standing position, with your legs about shoulder-distance apart. Bend your knees slightly. Grasp a toning stick or light dumbbell in each hand, with an overhand grip. Hold the weights at your thighs, with your palms facing toward you and your arms fully extended.

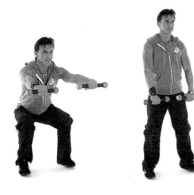

Action: Squat down so that your thighs are parallel to the floor. As you squat, lift the weights straight up in front of you, as shown.

Straighten your legs as your arms return to the starting position. Repeat the move for a series of repetitions.

Zumba Lateral Travel

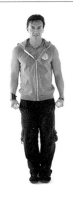

Start: In this move, you will take two steps to the side, while lifting the weights up and to the side in a special sequence.

First, let's get a sense of how to lift the toning sticks or a pair of light dumbbells in this sequence. The move goes like this: Stand with your feet together and hold the weights in each hand held at your sides.

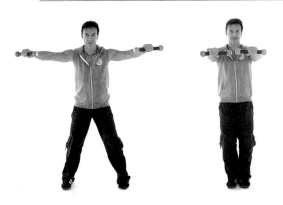

Keeping your elbows slightly bent, raise the weights up from your sides to a shoulder-level position as you step right into a wide-stance position. This is the "open" position.

From there, bring your arms together in front of you, at about chest level, as you bring your feet back together. This the "close" position.

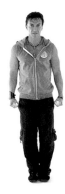

Next, lower your arms to your sides. This is the "down" position.

The arm sequence thus goes like this: open, close, down; open, close, down; and so forth.

Action: Once you get the hang of that, combine it with the leg movement. Here goes: Step to your right and lift the weights up to your sides (open). Bring your left foot to your right foot, closing the position, as you close your arms in front of you (close), then bring them down (down).

Step a second time to your right, repeating the same sequence with your arms. Repeat this entire move twice to your right. Switch sides and move twice to the left. You will really feel this move in your arms and shoulders.

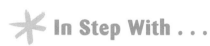

✳ In Step With . . .

Linda Hillsman, La Grange Park, Illinois

More than five years ago, Linda Hillsman, a shy mother of three, had just finished chemotherapy and radiation for breast cancer when she headed to Miami to become licensed as a Zumba instructor. Her goal was not just to obtain her license, but to help others become the best they can be through Zumba.

"Since then, I've had so many people approach me after class and thank me for helping them feel better about themselves, helping them relieve stress, helping them lose weight, and creating a 'family' atmosphere in class," she says. "I, too, can say the same thing. I am six years post–cancer treatment. I feel better and look stronger than I have in years."

Being a Zumba instructor has spilled over into Linda's life in other ways. One of her daughters is on the local high school Pom & Dance team. Sometimes mother and daughter dance together in the kitchen. Even Linda's son dances alongside her while she's learning new routines from Zumba Fitness DVDs.

"Zumba has changed my life and has been a positive influence on my children. I'm more confident and I feel I have a positive influence on the people in my class."

Linda has great advice for anyone doing Zumba Fitness: "Get outside your comfort zone. Just relax and let go. Shake your shoulders and relieve your stress. Listen to the music and let your mind travel to your favorite warm and sunny place. Most of all, have fun, drink plenty of water, burn calories, and feel strong."

ZUMBA BUNS AND THIGHS

To work the lower body, I love to incorporate moves borrowed from flamenco, the traditional song and dance of southern Spain. Flamenco is considered a unique fusion of native Arabic, Islamic, and gypsy cultures. This centuries-old rhythm incorporates instruments like the guitar, violin, flute, bass, and various percussion items as vehicles for expression, capable of depicting soft and sweet emotions as well as anger and strength. Much of this intense feeling comes out not just through the steps and live musical accompaniment, but through the moves dancers make with their hands and feet. Some say, "People don't watch flamenco, they feel it."

Flamenco fitness dancing can be a high-calorie-burning workout because it brings into play a variety of large muscle groups. It typically involves deep lunges, stretching, fast-paced walking, and jumping—so you can see why it is great for your thighs and buns.

ZUMBA FITNESS TIP:
4 Ways to Spice Up Your Workouts

* Stay in the moment when you do Zumba and you will get better results. Staying focused helps you dance and move to your full potential.

* If you have any joint problems, take a warm shower before you do Zumba. The shower will loosen up your joints.

* Chart your progress. Mark down each time you work out, and how many minutes you exercised. Keep your chart on your fridge as a reminder of how well you are doing.

* Make a date. Treat Zumba as a social time by pairing up with a friend or your spouse to go to a class. If you commit to someone else, you will be less likely to skip your workout.

Flamenco Knee Lift

Start: Stand tall, with your feet together and your hands on your hips.

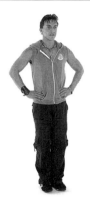

Action: Beginning on your right foot, take a step on the ball of your foot.

Then return to a flat step.

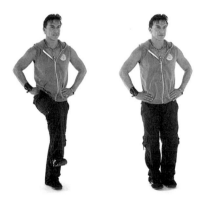

Next, do the same on your left foot. Step again on your right foot. Then raise your right knee as high as you can in front of your torso.

The sequence is thus: right step, flat; left step, flat; right step, lift, then down. Repeat the sequence, this time leading with your left foot.

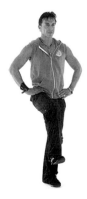

Flamenco Side Lunges

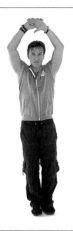

Start: Begin with your feet together and your arms overhead with "attitude," as shown.

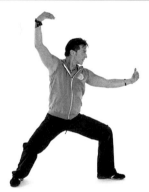

Action: Keeping your back as straight as possible, step sideways with your left foot as far as you can until your thigh is just about parallel to the floor.

Your right arm remains up, and your left is extended. This is what I call "flamenco arms."

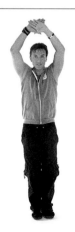

Press back to the starting position and return your arms to the overhead position.

Do the lunge on your left leg. Alternate for a series of repetitions.

Flamenco Squats

Start: Begin with your feet together and your arms overhead with "attitude," as shown.

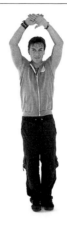

Action: Keeping your back as straight as possible, step sideways with your right foot. Squat so that both thighs are just about parallel to the floor.

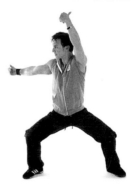

Return to the starting position and repeat for a series of repetitions.

Repeat on your left side.

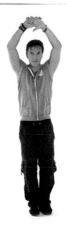

Zumba Bun Tightener

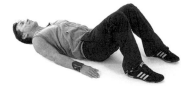

Start: Lie on your back on a mat or soft carpet. Place your hands at your side. Your feet should be on the floor and your knees bent.

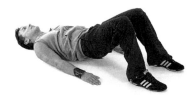

Action: Lift your glutes off the floor as high as you can and squeeze them together.

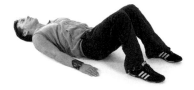

Lower your glutes back to the floor.

Try for ten repetitions if you are new to exercise or out of condition; and twenty to thirty if you have been exercising for a while.

Spice It Up: As you lift your glutes, open your knees. Then close your knees and squeeze your glutes. Lower back to the floor.

ZUMBA TOTAL BODY STRETCHES

After any Zumba workout, I like to flow into a slow stretching session where the rhythms sound relaxing, the heart rate can return to normal, and we are ready to end the sessions with a more relaxed mind and body. I end the session with long, slow, static stretching. The muscles are warm enough now to accept such stretches, about ten seconds per stretch. This is the cool-down portion of the Zumba workout.

A cool-down consisting of a gradual reduction in exercise intensity is highly recommended following any workout. A cool-down provides multiple benefits. It allows a gradual reduction in heart rate and cardiac output, provides the blood vessels in the legs a chance to constrict back toward their original diameter, and the dynamic action of the contracting muscles prevents any pooling of blood in the legs. (If you stop exercising suddenly, your blood may pool in the extremities, causing dizziness, nausea, or cramping.)

This all works together to bring blood flow, blood pressure, and body temperature from the high levels encountered during exercise gradually back down toward resting levels. It is also the time to stretch your muscles for flexibility, as well as to reduce soreness and prevent cramping or injury, and transition from large muscle movements to smaller muscle movements.

Perform the following five-minute stretching routine after your Zumba workouts. Be sure to breathe deeply, never holding your breath.

And continue the fun by cooling down to music! Choose songs such as a flamenco or tango for your cool-down—songs that are slow and mellow.

Lower Leg and Upper Hip Stretch

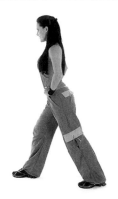

Start: Stand in a lunge position with your right foot forward and left foot back, toes pointed straight ahead. Place your hands on your right thigh or on a sturdy chair for support.

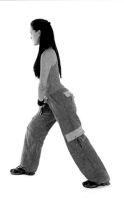

Action: Bend your right knee and lunge forward, keeping your left leg straight and your torso upright.

Press both hips forward until you feel a stretch in the front of your left hip and the back of your left lower leg. Hold for 10 seconds, release, and repeat 5 more times. Switch sides and repeat.

Side Torso Stretch

Start: Stand tall with your arms reaching straight above your head, hands clasped, and abs pulled in.

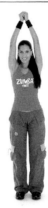

Action: Inhale, then exhale as you lean to the left, feeling a stretch in the right side of your torso. Hold for 10 seconds.

Return to center.

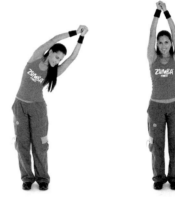

Then repeat on the opposite side. Repeat 5 times on each side.

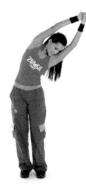

Low-Back Stretch

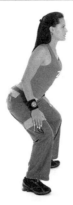

Start: Stand with your feet hip-width apart, knees bent, and hands on your upper thighs.

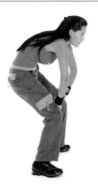

Action: Inhale, then exhale as you draw in your abs and round your back, curling your tailbone under you and tucking your chin toward your chest. You should feel the stretch in your lower back.

Hold for 10 seconds, then release. Repeat 5 times.

 In Step With . . .

Vanessa Lupercio, Mesa, Arizona

Vanessa Lupercio, 33, will tell you that discovering Zumba was a turning point in her life. The mother of two children, she recalled that losing her maternity weight seemed impossible. Vanessa tried Zumba, loved it, and kept at it. She lost twenty-two pounds in about twelve weeks, and firmed up all her trouble spots. She was hooked.

"It's an amazing program," she said of Zumba. "It targets hips, thighs, abs—and it's having fun, having a good time! You have a great time, feel beautiful, and you walk out of there with a whole new attitude. You can't get that from an elliptical machine."

Total Body Stretch

Start: Position yourself on a mat or soft carpet in an all-fours crouching position.

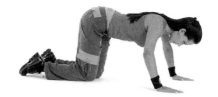

Action: Inhale, then exhale as you begin to lift your hips and straighten your arms and legs, coming into an inverted V position (also known as "downward facing dog" in yoga).

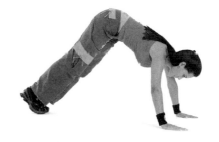

Hold for 10 seconds, breathing deeply and feeling a stretch in the back of your legs, calves, chest, shoulders, and sides of your torso.

Bend your knees and release them to the floor, then sit back onto your heels with your arms on the floor and your chest resting on your thighs to stretch your lower back and shoulders.

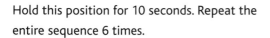

Hold this position for 10 seconds. Repeat the entire sequence 6 times.

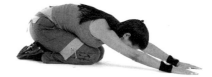

Low Back and Hip Stretch

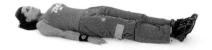

Start: Lie on your back on a mat or soft carpet with your legs straight out in front of you.

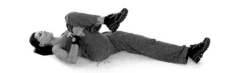

Action: Bend your right knee, grasp the back of your thigh, and bring your knee in toward your chest. Hold for 10 seconds.

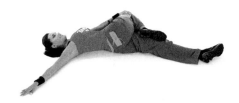

Then, using your left hand, bring your right knee across your body and down toward the floor. Look over your right shoulder and reach your right arm out to the side, keeping your right shoulder in contact with the floor.

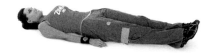

Hold for 10 seconds, feeling a stretch in your lower back and hip. Release and come to center, then switch sides. Repeat the sequence 5 times on each side.

After a Zumba sculpt, tone, and stretch workout, I feel invigorated, sweaty, and completely energized. It is the perfect workout when you desire something different, where the emphasis is on having fun.

Chapter 7

BURN FAT, HAVE FUN: THE AT-HOME ZUMBA ROUTINES

Zumba is exercise *and* dance, so let the entertainer in you come shimmying out onto the exercise floor. We all want to be stars—and here is your chance to do it. You have already learned the basic steps, along with my sculpting moves and stretches; now you are ready to party! With the routines I have created for you in this chapter and in the enclosed DVD, you can work out in the convenience of your own home.

THE ZUMBA DVD WORKOUTS

In this chapter and on the DVD, you will find three twenty-minute Zumba workouts. You can perform them consecutively to create an hour-long workout. Or if you are tight on time, or new to Zumba and want to pick up the basics, you can do one of the twenty-minute workouts by itself.

THE ZUMBA SCULPT AND TONE WORKOUT

If you want to concentrate on your "trouble spots" such as abs, thighs, or buns, this workout shows you how. It combines the sculpting moves and stretches you learned in Chapter 6 for a targeted workout focusing on muscle strength and shaping. You can do this workout alone, or tack it on to the end of one of the twenty-minute workouts for additional calorie-burning and bodyshaping.

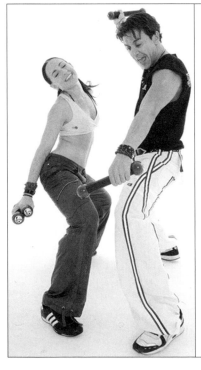

For a Safe Zumba Workout at Home

✳ Clear a large area in your home to give yourself room to dance. Move furniture, lift the rugs, and relocate breakable objects so you can kick up your feet and have enough space around you for full range of motion of your arms and legs.

✳ Keep the temperature in the room between 65 and 75 degrees Fahrenheit—warm enough to let you sweat, yet cool enough to feel comfortable and not overheated.

✳ Dance with a sense of abandon. No one is watching, so forget self-consciousness and get lost in the beat.

✳ Even though you may get hooked on Zumba and want to do more, it is a good idea to schedule one, two, or three days of rest from Zumba in your week, especially as you start out. "Recovery" days are important to let your body rebuild. They also let you push harder on workout days.

MATCHING THE MOVES TO MUSIC:
HOW THE 20-MINUTE WORKOUTS ARE STRUCTURED

In Zumba routines, different dance moves are matched to different parts of a song, so it helps to know how songs are typically put together. Musicians group their songs according to the following components:

Intro: The first part of a song before the verse or chorus begins.

Verse: This part is usually the "story" or "talking" part of a song. Usually, a verse occurs two to three times in a song. The musical part is the same each time, but often the words are different.

Chorus: The chorus is a line or group of lines repeated at intervals in a song. It generally incorporates the same words (and the same musical part) each time it is played. The title of the song is often repeated in the chorus.

Break, Bridge, Tag, Musical Interludes: These are pieces and parts of a song that are not part of the verse or the chorus. They might be pauses (breaks) in a song, a bridge between parts, a musical segment, or an unusual set of beats.

When broken into its components, a song might look like this: Intro—Verse—Chorus—Verse—Chorus—Tag—Verse—Chorus—Tag—Chorus. With this kind of structure, it is easy to follow along with the music.

As you perform the routine to the DVD, you will notice that there is a timer on the screen. Each series of moves is timed. So when the time is up for one move, that is your cue that a new move begins.

As you learn the routines on the DVD, I encourage you to add variety and style. I love not only bringing my personal style into the workout, but encouraging my class members to develop their own style. In addition to doing only three or four basic moves, you can add arm, directional, or fitness variations to spice them up. Feel the emotional quality of the music, and move to it—and let your heart beat to all of it. And practice! The more you practice, the better your routine will be.

Now, for the routines. *Uno, dos, tres—vamanos!* (One, two, three—let's go!)

Routine #1

Total Time: 20 minutes

Effort: Try to work in the RPE zones of at least 3–4.

SALSA

Music: "Zumbando Al Son" (5:31)

RHYTHM	FROM:	TO:
1. Cuban Step (step right, close; step left, close)	0:00	0:52
2. Basic Salsa	0:52	1:22
3. Cuban Step (shimmy your shoulders)	1:22	1:30
4. Cuban Step	1:30	1:39
5. Basic Salsa	1:39	2:08
6. Cuban Step with fitness variation	2:08	2:25
7. Salsa Back Step (step back right, close; step back left, close)	2:25	2:40
8. Basic Salsa	2:40	3:15
9. Salsa Back Step (step back right, close; step back left, close)	3:15	3:32
10. Basic Salsa	3:32	4:03
11. Salsa Back Step (step back right, close; step back left, close)	4:03	4:19
12. Basic Salsa	4:19	4:39
13. Basic Salsa	4:39	5:02
14. Cuban Step with fitness variation	5:02	5:31

CUMBIA

Music: "Cumbia Jam" (4:02)

RHYTHM	FROM:	TO:
1. Sway your hips to the music	0:00	0:10
2. Basic Cumbia to the right	0:10	0:22
3. Basic Cumbia to the left	0:22	0:34
4. Basic Cumbia to the right	0:34	0:46
5. Sleepy Leg to the right in a circle	0:46	0:56
6. Sleepy Leg to the left in a circle	0:56	1:06
7. Sugar cane to the right	1:06	1:37
8. Sway your hips to the music	1:37	2:09
9. Basic Cumbia to the left	2:09	2:21
10. Basic Cumbia to the right	2:21	2:32
11. Basic Cumbia to the left	2:32	2:44
12. Sleepy Leg to the right in a circle	2:44	2:54
13. Sleepy Leg to the left in a circle	2:54	3:04
14. Sugar Cane to the left	3:04	3:34
15. Booty Circle to the right	3:34	3:48
16. Squats	3:48	4:02

REGGAETON

Music: "Mira La" (4:55)

RHYTHM	FROM:	TO:
1. Basic Reggaeton	0:00	0:27
2. Reggaeton Bounce	0:27	1:05
3. Basic Reggaeton with variation (single, single, double)	1:05	1:14
4. Reggaeton Bounce	1:14	1:41
5. Basic Reggaeton with variation (single, single, double)	1:41	1:58
6. Reggaeton Stomp	1:58	2:07
7. Reggaeton Bounce	2:07	2:25
8. Reggaeton Stomp	2:25	2:33
9. Basic Reggaeton with variation (single, single, double)	2:33	2:51
10. Reggaeton Stomp	2:51	3:09
11. Reggaeton Bounce	3:09	3:19
12. Reggaeton Stomp	3:19	3:36
13. Basic Reggaeton with variation (single, single, double)	3:36	3:53
14. Reggaeton Stomp	3:53	4:20
15. Basic Reggaeton with variation (single, single, double)	4:20	4:55

Routine #2

Total Time: 20 minutes

Effort: Try to work in the RPE zones of at least 3–4.

MERENGUE

Music: "Quien Baila, Quien Goza" (5:12)

RHYTHM	FROM:	TO:
1. Merengue March (march in place; let your arms move naturally)	0:00	1:16
2. Side-to-Side Merengue (2 steps to the right, 2 steps to the left)	1:16	1:30
3. Side-to-Side Merengue with fitness (2 steps to the right—lunge; 2 steps to the left—lunge)	1:30	1:45
4. Beto Shuffle	1:45	1:59
5. Side-to-Side Merengue with fitness (2 steps to the right—lunge; 2 steps to the left—lunge)	1:59	2:29
6. Beto Shuffle	2:29	2:55
7. Side-to-Side Merengue	2:55	3:10
8. Side-to-Side Merengue with fitness (2 steps to the right—lunge; 2 steps to the left—lunge)	3:10	3:22
9. Beto Shuffle	3:22	3:36
10. Side-to-Side Merengue	3:36	4:16
11. Beto Shuffle	4:16	4:43
12. Side-to-Side Merengue with fitness (2 steps to the right—lunge; 2 steps to the left—lunge)	4:43	5:12

SALSA

Music: "Ya Llego" (4:55)

RHYTHM	FROM:	TO:
1. Touch your toes to the front, first your right toe, then left toe, alternating in this fashion	0:00	0:26
2. Basic Salsa	0:26	0:43
3. Cuban Step	0:43	1:01
4. Salsa Back Step	1:01	1:18
5. Cuban Step with fitness	1:18	1:33
6. Touch your toes to the front, first your right toe, then left toe, alternating in this fashion	1:33	1:51
7. Basic Salsa	1:51	2:08
8. Cuban Step	2:08	2:26
9. Touch your toes to the front, first your right toe, then left toe, alternating in this fashion	2:26	2:35
10. Cuban Step with arm variation	2:35	3:13
11. Salsa Back Step	3:13	3:30
12. Cuban Step with fitness	3:30	3:45
13. Touch your toes to the front, first your right toe, then left toe, alternating in this fashion	3:45	4:03
14. Salsa Back Step	4:03	4:20
15. Cuban Step with fitness	4:20	4:36
16. Touch your toes to the front, first your right toe, then left toe, alternating in this fashion	4:36	4:55

CUMBIA

Music: "Santa Que" (6:05)

RHYTHM	FROM:	TO:
1. Sway your hips to the music	0:00	0:30
2. Sway your hips to the music; add claps	0:30	0:49
3. Basic Cumbia to the right	0:49	1:11
4. Sugar Cane to the right	1:11	1:40
5. Sugar Cane to the left	1:40	2:01
6. Sleepy Leg to the right in a circle	2:01	2:20
7. Sleepy Leg to the right in a circle	2:20	2:40
8. Reggaeton Stomp	2:40	3:00
9. Sleepy leg to the right in a circle	3:00	3:17
10. Sugar Cane to the left	3:17	3:35
11. Sway your hips to the music	3:35	3:45
12. Sleepy Leg to the left in a circle	3:45	4:04
13. Sway your hips to the music	4:04	4:10
14. Sleepy Leg to the right in a circle	4:10	4:30
15. Sugar Cane to the right	4:30	4:56
16. Basic Cumbia to the left	4:56	5:26
17. Sleepy Leg to the right in a circle	5:26	5:44
18. Reggaeton Stomp	5:44	6:05

REGGAETON

Music: "Zumbalicious" (4:25)

RHYTHM	FROM:	TO:
1. Basic Reggaeton	0:00	0:10
2. Reggaeton Bounce	0:10	0:20
3. Reggaeton Stomp	0:20	0:30
4. Reggaeton Bounce	0:30	0:39
5. Reggaeton Stomp	0:39	0:49
6. Reggaeton Bounce	0:49	1:00
7. Reggaeton Stomp	1:00	1:10
8. Reggaeton Bounce	1:10	1:20
9. Reggaeton Stomp	1:20	1:30
10. Reggaeton Bounce	1:30	1:39
11. Booty Circle to the right	1:39	1:49
12. Basic Reggaeton with variation (single, single, double)	1:49	2:07
13. Basic Reggaeton with variation (single, single, double); add arm variation	2:07	2:18
14. Reggaeton Stomp	2:18	2:28
15. Reggaeton Bounce	2:28	2:38
16. Reggaeton Stomp	2:38	2:47
17. Reggaeton Bounce	2:47	2:57
18. Reggaeton Stomp	2:57	3:07
19. Reggaeton Bounce	3:07	3:17
20. Reggaeton Stomp	3:17	3:27
21. Reggaeton Bounce	3:27	3:36
22. Basic Reggaeton with variation (single, single, double)	3:36	4:25

Routine #3

Total Time: 20 minutes

Effort: Try to work in the RPE zones of at least 3–4.

MERENGUE

Music: "Que Te Mueve" (5:08)

RHYTHM	FROM:	TO:
1. Merengue March (march in place; let your arms move naturally)	0:00	0:36
2. Side-to-Side Merengue (2 steps to the right, 2 steps to the left)	0:36	0:51
3. March 4 steps to the side and jump when you hear the clap	0:51	1:05
4. March 4 steps to each side	1:05	1:21
5. Beto Shuffle	1:21	1:50
6. Side-to-Side Merengue	1:50	2:20
7. Booty Circle to the right	2:20	2:34
8. Booty Circle to the left	2:34	2:49
9. March 4 steps to each side	2:49	3:04
10. Shimmy to the music: Take a wide stance and shimmy your shoulders and hips, while holding your arms out to the side at shoulder level.	3:04	3:12
11. Shake your hips and your chest from side to side	3:12	3:53
12. March 4 steps to each side	3:53	4:08
13. Side-to-Side Merengue	4:08	4:23
14. March 4 steps to each side	4:23	4:38
15. Beto Shuffle	4:38	5:08

SALSA

Music: "Zumbando Por Un Sueno" (4:34)

RHYTHM	FROM:	TO:
1. Move your hips from side to side to the trumpet sound	0:00	0:10
2. Touch your toes to the front, first your right toe, then left toe, alternating in this fashion	0:10	0:39
3. Move your hips from side to side	0:39	0:49
4. Basic Salsa	0:49	0:58
5. Salsa Back Step	0:58	1:18
6. Cuban Step	1:18	1:38
7. Salsa Back Step	1:38	2:07
8. Cuban Step	2:07	2:26
9. Cuban Step with fitness	2:26	2:36
10. Basic Salsa	2:36	2:56
11. Reggaeton Stomp	2:56	3:25
12. Cuban Step	3:25	3:45
13. Move your hips from side to side to the trumpet sound	3:45	3:55
14. Reggaeton Stomp	3:55	4:15
15. Salsa Back Step	4:15	4:34

CUMBIA

Music: "Zumba Kumbia" (4:25)

RHYTHM	FROM:	TO:
1. Sway your hips to the music.	0:00	0:20
2. Basic Cumbia to the right	0:20	0:29
3. Basic Cumbia to the left	0:29	0:38
4. Sleepy Leg to the right	0:38	0:48
5. Sleepy Leg to the left	0:48	0:58
6. Sugar Cane to the right	0:58	1:18
7. Sleepy Leg to the left	1:18	1:28
8. Basic Cumbia to the right	1:28	1:37
9. Basic Cumbia to the left	1:37	1:47
10. Sugar Cane to the left	1:47	2:02
11. Sleepy Leg to the right	2:02	2:11
12. Sleepy Leg to the left	2:11	2:21
13. Basic Cumbia to the right	2:21	2:31
14. Basic Cumbia to the right in a circle	2:31	2:40
15. Sleepy Leg to the right	2:40	2:50
16. Sleepy Leg to the left	2:50	3:05
17. Sugar Cane to the right	3:05	3:43
18. Basic Cumbia to the right	3:43	3:52
19. Sugar Cane to the left	3:52	4:02
20. Sleepy Leg to the right	4:02	4:11
21. Basic Cumbia to the right	4:11	4:25

REGGAETON

Music: "Muevete Pa' Aca Muevete Pa' Alla" (4:13)

RHYTHM	FROM:	TO:
1. Basic Reggaeton	0:00	0:25
2. Basic Reggaeton (single, single, double)	0:25	0:43
3. Reggaeton Bounce	0:43	1:06
4. Basic Reggaeton (single, single, double)	1:06	1:40
5. Reggaeton Stomp	1:40	1:57
6. Reggaeton Bounce	1:57	2:22
7. Basic Reggaeton (single, single, double)	2:22	2:54
8. Beto Shuffle	2:54	3:20
9. Reggaeton Stomp	3:20	3:40
10. Basic Reggaeton (single, single, double)	3:40	4:13

Cool-Down

* Take a wide stance and shimmy your shoulders for 30 to 45 seconds. This belly-dancing move involves holding your arms gently out at shoulder level and pushing the right shoulder forward as the left goes back. Reverse the shoulder positions, pushing the left shoulder forward as the right goes back. Repeat the alternation, gradually increasing the speed.

* Side torso stretch; once to the right, once to the left.

* Take your body down to a squat; roll back up, one vertebra at a time.

* Inhale, reaching up to ceiling with your arms; exhale, bringing your arms back down. Repeat.

Beto's Comments

If you would like to get some extra exercise in, perform my Sculpt & Tone Workout (see next page), right after this workout but prior to the cool-down. Afterward, you can cool down by using the instructions on this page. Or you have the option of doing my Total Body Stretches as your cool-down.

The Zumba Sculpt & Tone Workout

Warm-Up: To prepare your body for this workout, I suggest doing the Merengue March, the Side-to-Side Merengue, and the Beto Shuffle. These moves will warm your body up.

Total Time: 20–25 minutes

Suggested Music: Any slow-tempo music that you enjoy.

Effort: Try to work in the RPE zones of at least 3–4

AB EXERCISES	REPETITIONS	SETS
Booty Circle	8 full circles	2–4
Reggaeton Crunch	8 times right knee, 8 times left knee	2–4
Zumba Standing Twist	Left, right—8 times	2–4
Urban Core Twist	20 times	2–4
UPPER BODY EXERCISES	**REPETITIONS**	**SETS**
Zumba Curls with light weights or toning sticks	15	2–4
Zumba Triceps Press with light weights or toning sticks	15	2–4
Zumba Overhead Press with light weights or toning sticks	15	2–4
Zumba Lateral Raise & Squat with light weights or toning sticks	15	2–4
Zumba Lateral Travel with light weights or toning sticks	10 times to the right; 10 times to the left	2–4
LOWER BODY EXERCISES	**REPETITIONS**	**SETS**
Flamenco Knee Lifts	Alternate right/left knees for a total of 20 times	2–4
Flamenco Side Lunge	10 times to the right; 10 times to the left	2–4
Flamenco Squat	10 squats on the right; 10 squats on the left	2–4
Zumba Bun Tightener	15	2–4

Cool-Down: Perform my Total Body Stretches (see pages 125–130).

Beto's Comments

As you perform these body-sculpting moves, be sure to think about the muscle group you are working. The more you force the muscle or muscle group to contract (flex), the more you will benefit. Move through these exercises slowly and deliberately, without momentum doing the work for you. With squats and lunges, keep your knees over your toes, your core muscles tight, and your back erect. For added intensity, do not be afraid to increase the amount of weight you do, the number of repetitions or sets you perform, or both. The more you push yourself (without overdoing it), the more fat you will burn and the more toned your body will become.

A FITTER, FIRMER BODY IN NINE WEEKS

Generally, your body changes and adapts to regular exercise in three-week cycles. This means you will want to change your routine every three weeks, gradually increasing how many workouts you do (frequency) and how long you do them (duration).

Here is a closer look at how to progress, based on whether you are a beginner, intermediate, or advanced exerciser.

Groovin' and Moving: The Beginner's Schedule

If you are just starting Zumba and have not done much aerobics-type exercise in the past, you will probably feel most comfortable doing one of the twenty-minute routines two to three times a week. After exercising at the beginner level for at least three weeks, move up to the intermediate option explained below.

Weeks 1–3

Day 1:   Routine 1, 2, or 3
Day 2:   Free Day
Day 3:   Routine 1, 2, or 3
Day 4:   Free Day
Day 5:   Routine 1, 2, or 3
Day 6:   Free Day
Day 7:   Routine 1, 2, or 3

Beto's Comments

You can definitely burn a quite a few calories by working out at home. If you opt to participate in hour-long Zumba classes, expect to burn even more—up to 1,000 calories an hour, depending on how much oomph you put into the class!

Bring the Party Up: The Intermediate Schedule

Here is where you can start transforming your shape and get super-sculpted—by combining the routines with the Sculpt & Tone Workout during the week.

Weeks 4–6

Day 1:   Zumba Sculpt & Tone followed by Total Body Stretch
Day 2:   Routine 1, 2, or 3
Day 3:   Zumba Sculpt & Tone followed by Total Body Stretch
Day 4:   Free Day
Day 5:   Routine 1, 2, or 3
Day 6:   Zumba Sculpt & Tone followed by Total Body Stretch
Day 7:   Routine 1, 2, or 3

Get the Most from Your Zumba Workout

Save Bigger Meals for Later. Do not have a heavy meal right before your workout. Rather, have a small, high-energy snack such as a piece of fresh fruit, yogurt, or a nutrition drink or bar.

Clear Your Mind. Before you start, mentally put aside any concerns, worries, or issues. Most people find Zumba to be a stress reliever. Use your workout to relax, clear your mind, and concentrate on your dancing.

Be Sensitive to Your Body. Always listen to your body. If you feel like you should not do that deep lunge, you probably should not attempt it.

Stay in the Moment. Emphasize fully experiencing Zumba while you are doing it. Enjoy what you look like, savor the flow while it happens, tune into the feeling of it, and express the music.

Have Fun. The most important part is to have fun. Try not worry about how you're moving. Now is not the time to be self-conscious. Enjoy yourself!

Turn Up the Heat: The Advanced Schedule

If you were doing aerobics-type exercise prior to picking up this book, you should be able to handle more workouts a week. Or if you have been exercising at the intermediate option for at least three weeks, you are also ready for more. With this routine, you can mix things up throughout the week, do some heart-pumping cardio training, body sculpting, and resistance moves.

Weeks 7–9

Day 1:   Routines 1, 2, and 3 (60 minutes) followed by Total Body Stretch

Day 2:   Zumba Sculpt & Tone followed by Total Body Stretch

Day 3:   Routines 1, 2, and 3 (60 minutes) followed by Total Body Stretch

Day 4:   Free Day

Day 5:   Zumba Sculpt & Tone followed by Total Body Stretch

Day 6:   Routines 1, 2, and 3 (60 minutes) followed by Total Body Stretch

Day 7:   Zumba Sculpt & Tone followed by Total Body Stretch

So there you have it—the routines and exercise schedule that will help you shed pounds, define muscles, and feel wonderful. But there's more: Every party has food, which is why I now want to introduce you to the Zumba Diet.

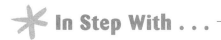 ## ✳ In Step With . . .

Karin Silvio, Philadelphia, Pennsylvania

Ask Karin about Zumba, and she'll tell you, "It has been life-changing for me."

At age forty-four, Karin decided to become a personal trainer and fitness instructor—which led her to get licensed to teach Zumba Fitness in 2008. Her classes grew larger and larger, while her enthusiastic students got smaller and more trim. "Everyone leaves class happy," she says.

The most rewarding part of her involvement with Zumba Fitness is that it has inspired her two teenage daughters, Barb, 18, and Riana, 16, not only to get fit, but also to know that if they put their minds to something, like their mom did, they can accomplish anything.

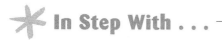 **In Step With . . .**

Alicia Burk, Pittsburg, Kansas

Alicia had a shelf full of fitness videos, some of which she had viewed only once and many others that still had the plastic wrap on them.

But after seeing an infomercial for Zumba Fitness one day, Alicia sensed there was something very different about it. "This was an exercise program that I knew I would like and could stick to. I immediately placed my order and could hardly wait for the DVDs to come in the mail. I had never felt that way about buying an exercise video in the past."

As soon as she got her new DVDs, Alicia popped them in the machine and, though sitting on the couch, she started dancing in her seat. "Before the end of the song, I was up on my feet and doing the salsa!

"Zumba was the first-ever exercise program that I enjoyed doing over and over. It is absolutely infectious. When the second collection came out, I immediately ordered them as well."

Eventually, Alicia sold or gave away all her other fitness videos. The Zumba Fitness DVDs are the only ones she owns. In no time at all, Alicia's jeans were fitting better. She lost forty-five pounds, a victory she calls "the easiest weight I've ever lost and kept off. The moves have done wonders for my waistline and more for my self-esteem. Everything on my body has toned, tightened, and lifted up! I never thought of myself as a dancer, but now I love to go dancing and show off the moves I've learned!"

Alicia has been attending Zumba classes for five years, and she still loves it as much as she did the day she played her first DVD. Sometimes she does Zumba twice a day. She and her girlfriends have organized Zumba parties, in which they congregate in her garage and dance all evening long.

"Spending time with my friends has never been so much fun! For that matter, exercising has never been so much fun! You don't have to know how to dance or already be in good shape to start and enjoy Zumba. I am happier, more confident, and in the best shape of my life thanks to Zumba."

Part Three

DITCH BORING DIETS: LET'S EAT TO BURN BELLY FAT AND THIGH FAT

Chapter 8
BODYSHAPING FOODS

Welcome, everyone, to the Zumba Diet. This is one of the most unique diets of its kind because it emphasizes "bodyshaping foods," foods that have been shown in scientific studies to target certain parts of the body, such as abs and thighs, and remove fat from those areas, as well as from the rest of your body. In fact, the Zumba Diet is really four diets in one: The Zumba 5-Day Express Diet, which can melt off up to nine pounds in five days; the Zumba Flat Abs Diet, to pry loose stubborn belly fat; the Zumba Thin Thighs Diet, with foods that target lower-body fat; and the Zumba Basic Diet for overall fat-burning. You can choose to follow any of these diets, depending on your bodyshaping goals. As you go forward on this plan, expect to experience at least ten great benefits:

* Slenderized, firm hips and thighs

* Flatter abs

* Better proportions

* Loss of inches

* Steady, satisfying weight loss

* Improved fitness

* Ample energy

* Greater self-confidence

* Positive feelings about yourself and your body

* Overall sense of well-being

The Zumba Diet will transform your figure in ways you never thought possible: You will have better proportions, less body fat, greater muscle tone and development, and more. It is all about maximizing your unique shape and looking fabulous. It is likely that you will feel so good after this program that you will decide to eat this way for the rest of your life. And before long, you will be able to bring back the contours in your body. Let me explain.

TARGETED DIETING

When you look at yourself in the mirror, it is not always your weight you dislike, but your shape. Maybe you'd like to change your hips or bottom if you are a woman, or perhaps the paunch or your skinny legs if you are a guy. Or you may feel out of proportion or not muscled enough. Whatever you look like, you would probably love to have a more defined and proportional shape.

If you just look around, you can see that body shape varies from person to person. There are several reasons why. First, your shape is largely determined by your genes—you take bits from both parents, but how you end up is a lottery. Second, your gender is also a key factor because each sex is genetically programmed with its own blueprint of muscle, bone, and fat. Guys have a lot more muscles than women, for example. Third, body shape varies among ethnic groups. For example, Asian adults are more prone to gain weight around the waist than Europeans are. Mediterranean women are prone to gain fat in the outer thighs. Fourth, there is the factor of lifestyle. Most people become softer and flabbier if they do not exercise and eat right, and of course this alters body shape.

Regular exercise definitely changes your body shape for the better. But did you know that certain foods have a direct bearing on where you carry fat and muscle on your body? It is a fact: researchers have discovered that there are foods that can actually affect your shape, plus promote overall weight loss. Isn't that amazing? These "bodyshaping" foods form the core of the Zumba Diet. For example, a number of foods target, and reduce, fat around the waistline; other foods target the lower body. Many foods are helpful for increasing lean muscle and/or decreasing overall body fat. (See the chart on the next page for an overview of bodyshaping foods.)

Using foods to enhance body shape is what we at Zumba Fitness call "targeted dieting." Never forget, though: You cannot change your shape without exercise. You need a combination of aerobic and resistance training to build a strong, attractive body, and Zumba provides that combination.

So at the heart of the Zumba Diet are nutritious foods that work with your body to enhance shape. And guess what else? These foods happen to be very healthy. They are foods everyone should be eating, every day. So in addition to improving your waistline and other parts of your body, you will be improving your health.

TARGETED DIETING: HOW FOOD AFFECTS BODY SHAPE

BODYSHAPING FOODS	HOW THEY WORK
Fiber-rich foods (whole grains, fruits, and vegetables)	Fiber helps reduce thigh fat when daily fiber levels average 26 grams. Scientists speculate that ample fiber helps escort excess estrogen from the body. Estrogen is partly responsible for laying down fat on the lower body, particularly in women.
Fish	Omega-3 fats in fish help reduce the size of fat cells in the body.
Monounsaturated fat (olive oil, canola oil, etc.)	This type of fat helps prevent body fat from congregating around the waistline.
Protein (fish, poultry, and lean meats)	Ample protein in the diet preserves lean muscle for a more efficient metabolism and better overall fat-burning; helps build and repair muscle; increases thermogenesis (a way the body burns excess food).
"Resistant starches" (beans, legumes, barley, etc.)	These special carbohydrates contain a unique type of dietary fiber that resists digestion. By replacing some of the normal starch with resistant starch, you burn up to 25 percent more fat over the course of the day.
Soy foods	Soy contains compounds that counter the action of fat-storing hormones in the body to prevent weight gain.
Calcium-rich foods	A high-calcium diet accelerates fat loss, particularly in the midsection. Why? Without enough calcium, the body produces a hormone called calcitriol, which sends a message to the fat cells telling them to store rather than release excess fat. Calcitriol seems to affect belly fat in particular by stimulating fat cells deep in the belly to produce cortisol, a hormone that instructs those cells to hang on to fat. Get an adequate amount of calcium, however, and you reverse the process.
Whole grains	Whole grains have been shown in research to reduce abdominal fat and overall body weight, whereas calories from refined grains (like white bread) tend to settle at the waist. Scientists do not know exactly why, but they think that refined grains are broken down more quickly into sugar. When sugars flood the body, insulin levels rise to help pull the sugars out of the bloodstream and store them in cells, often as fat.
Yogurt	When used with a low-calorie diet, yogurt helps decrease fat around the waistline due to yogurt's calcium content.

Source: Various studies published in scientific journals; see References section pages 285–287.

LOSE POUNDS AND INCHES
WITH BODYSHAPING FOODS

By incorporating bodyshaping foods, the Zumba Diet is set up to help you lose two to three pounds a week, especially if you are involved in a Zumba class or are exercising with Zumba at home. The diet supplies a combination of basic nutrients—protein, carbohydrate, fat, vitamins, minerals, and water—in amounts to help you improve your shape, lose weight, and feel energized.

The foods you eat are mostly natural and unprocessed, a type of eating for which the body is designed. You will feel full with just the right amount of food, and you will not be plagued by the enemy of dieting: hunger. As you become familiar with the food choices, you will find that the diet is simple to follow. And it will be fun to see your shape change.

To lose pounds and inches, you will need to eat fewer calories each day than you burn off. Calorie reduction plays a role in targeted dieting, too; cutting back on calories has also been found in research to help burn thigh fat, which is often difficult to lose. Even though the Zumba Diet reduces calories, you do not have to count calories or weigh out your servings. Everything is done for you.

You accelerate your weight loss by adding calorie-burning exercise to this equation through Zumba. Zumba expends additional calories, up to 600 to 1,000 calories an hour, depending on how hard you work out. What's more, you will be developing attractive, lean muscle, and muscle burns off more calories than do fatter bodies.

Proportionately, the Zumba Diet is higher in protein. Higher-protein diets stimulate fat-burning, particularly in the abdominal region of the body, and they help keep weight off after you have lost it. Protein also helps you develop body-flattering muscle.

In addition, the diet is neither too low nor too high in carbohydrates. It contains just the right amount that has been shown to promote steady weight loss. The Zumba Diet is also rich in fiber, a type of carb. Fibrous foods such as fruits, whole grains, and vegetables provide bulk. You thus feel full while eating a meal, so you are less tempted to overeat. High-fiber foods also take longer to chew, so your meals last longer. That is a plus, since it takes about twenty minutes after starting a meal for your body to send signals that it is full. And, when eaten with other nutrients like protein, fiber slows the rate of digestion, too, curbing your appetite between meals.

Finally, the diet is moderate in healthy fat. Moderate fat intake has been shown in research to help with weight loss and maintenance of weight loss—and to do so better than low-fat diets. Fat also has an appetite-suppressing effect.

Overall, a moderate-fat, moderate-carbohydrate, higher-protein diet is an excellent way to lose weight. You feel full and satisfied. You burn fat and preserve lean muscle. You feel highly energized throughout the day. For the most part, you are simply going to be healthier and in much better shape by following this type of plan.

 ## In Step With . . .

Josephine Grob, La Grange, Illinois

The year was 1995. Josephine Grob tried to squeeze herself into an airline seat and was horrified to discover that the seat belt would not fit around her waist. Too embarrassed to ask for a seat belt extender, she covered her lap with a sweater. Josephine was at her highest weight ever: 295 pounds. "That day was my rock bottom. I knew at that point that I had to change my life and take control of my eating and believe in myself."

Up until that fateful trip, Josephine had been a chronic dieter, starting a new diet one week and quitting it the next. "I felt so ugly, alone, and angry that I lost control over my eating habits. Food was my escape from reality; I ate large quantities of fatty foods every time my emotions took over. Every day, I would wake up thinking that today is the day my new diet begins, but I would never stick to it. I just hated looking in the mirror and not recognizing the person looking back at me. I was very big and unhappy, but that did not seem to stop the cycle of eating poorly."

That cycle included eating the following foods in a day, on average: five large pancakes with lots of syrup or an entire box of dry sugary cereal for breakfast; hamburger with fries and regular soda or two sandwiches with lots of mayonnaise and a large bag of chips for lunch; pizza or some type of fast food like tacos or fried rice with orange chicken for dinner; and ice cream, lots of candy bars, or a full box of cookies for snacks.

After returning from her trip, Josephine started a new diet and was determined to succeed. Her first move was to eliminate all junk food, cut out fatty foods, eat more fruits and vegetables, and keep a food journal to track her daily calories. Typically, a day's worth of meals included whole grains or low-carb pasta, fruits and vegetables, legumes, chicken or tuna, low-sugar snacks, and low-fat dairy foods—very similar to the Zumba Diet today.

"It was still difficult to work out, but I started walking outdoors for fifteen minutes a day until I was able to reach thirty minutes without feeling tired. It was imperative to exercise an average of four to five days a week in order to complete my new way of life by eating healthy and becoming fit."

Back then, Josephine's workout consisted of cardio four to five times a week, for up to forty-five minutes each time, along with strength training three days a week, for twenty to twenty-five minutes each session.

Her efforts paid off. She began losing two to three pounds a week, consistently. After the first six months, she had lost forty pounds and felt great about her accomplishment. In twenty-two months, Josephine lost a total of 145 pounds.

Propelled by her miraculous success, achieved entirely on her own, Josephine decided that she wanted to help other people achieve their own fitness goals.

In 2006, she became a licensed personal trainer and began teaching group exercise classes. The very next year, Josephine read about Zumba and took a workshop. "I have been teaching Zumba classes since January 2008 and absolutely love it. My students are having the time of their life and my classes are definitely growing.

"Never once did I imagine being in the fitness field and loving every minute of it. You can achieve any goal that you put your heart and soul into."

SPECIAL HEALTH BENEFITS OF THE ZUMBA DIET

First, let me say that I am not a nutritionist or a chef. I have no idea how many grams of fat are in a slice of cheese or how every single nutrient truly affects our bodies. But I am in a profession where people are concerned about weight and appearance, so I get a lot of questions from my students about how they can deal with their weight and get rid of extra pounds. Because of this, I stay on top of diet information. I do know what is healthy. I do know that it is important to eat more fruit and vegetables. I do know that if you have to unwrap it or take it out of a box, it is processed food and usually not good for your waistline or your health. That always seems to be the conclusion of most health advice we get, anyway.

The diet I grew up on—Latin cuisine—is very healthy, with a lot of healthy oils, fruits, vegetables, and lean proteins. So in this part of the book, we at Zumba Fitness are promoting healthy foods, and common-sense cooking, as a blueprint for losing weight. If you stick to this plan, you can enjoy food, have fun, lose weight, change your shape, and get healthier.

FEEL GREAT ON THE ZUMBA DIET

Zumba Diet is meant not just to help you lose weight and inches, but also to help you feel good, just as Zumba helps you feel good. For example, the diet is rich in fruits and vegetables. As soon as you start eating more of these foods, you should start feeling healthier. And no wonder: Studies show that a diet rich in plant-based foods can help you conquer obesity, prevent heart disease, lower your blood pressure, and cut your risk of cancer. This type of diet will also keep you looking younger (and living longer). Vegetables are a major source of antioxidants, which to your body means less cell damage from free radicals (nasty molecules implicated in the aging process), less damage to collagen (i.e., fewer wrinkles), and less damage to the internal organs (meaning they wear out more slowly). Expect to notice more immediate changes, too. Within just a few weeks of switching to more fruits and veggies, I bet people will tell you that you are glowing.

You get to enjoy other plant-based foods, such as whole grains. These foods are natural energy foods. People in the U.S. tend to eat mostly refined grains: bleached flour products such as white bread, cookies and cakes, and white rice, which have little or no fiber. Whole grains, like brown rice and whole-wheat bread, are unrefined and therefore more healthy.

These foods are a good source of carbohydrates. With all the bad press carbs have received in recent years, let me set the record straight: You must include unrefined carbohydrates in your daily diet. They are not at the root of obesity. Instead, they provide essential fuel for your brain, central nervous system, and muscles, and they provide nutrients that decrease risk for heart disease, diabetes, and cancer. Plus, because their fiber content helps you feel full (and carries waste products through your digestive tract more quickly) whole grains can help you to lose weight.

You can easily identify most whole grains. They are generally oval-shaped and range in color from light brown to dark brown. If a grain is white or has fewer than two grams of fiber per one-ounce serving, chances are it is refined and no longer a "whole" grain. A few whole grains you will be adding to your diet include brown and wild rice, barley, oats, quinoa, and bulgur wheat.

The Zumba Diet also supplies omega-3 fats, a type of "good fat" I am sure you have heard about. You can get adequate amounts by eating one serving of fish a few times a week. These are generally the darker-fleshed fish like salmon, tuna, and mackerel. You can also get your omega-3s from walnuts. Omega-3s keep your arteries cleaner, so eat more of these foods.

The Zumba Diet allows for other healthy fats. Americans tend to eat more of the bad fat that clogs arteries and raises "bad" cholesterol: saturated fat, derived mostly from animal sources like red meat and dairy; and trans fats, formed from the partial hydrogenation of vegetable oils and found in margarine, french fries, and packaged foods like chips and cookies. If you eat big, fat-laden meals, blood gathers in the blood vessels near your stomach to help in the digestive process, so less of it gets to your muscles and brain, making you feel more sluggish.

The Zumba Diet emphasizes healthy fats like monounsaturated fats such as olive, canola, and flaxseed oil, as well as avocados and almonds, which reduce your LDL cholesterol (the bad kind), boost your HDL cholesterol, and help burn fat from your belly.

The diet minimizes refined sugar and junk food—the stuff that is largely responsible for obesity. Once you get it out of your system, you will start craving healthy food, and in the process, get rid of fat and reshape your body.

PREPARING FOR THE ZUMBA DIET

Getting in really great shape is a long-term commitment. You cannot join a Zumba group, work out for a couple of weeks, start a diet, and expect to be in tip-top shape right away. But the fact that you are reading this book indicates that you want to improve your life by developing a healthier body.

The toughest part is getting started. The second toughest part is staying motivated. It is a head game. So talk to yourself, give yourself encouragement, and love your body. It is crying out to be fit, and all it takes is a mere hour of exercise three days a week, along with a healthy diet, to get it into shape. Recognize the broader implications of diet and exercise—not just for staying lean and looking good, but for reducing the risk of disease and increasing your energy. Once you begin to take charge of your own well-being, "diet" and "sweat" will become beautiful words, and you will be well on your way to a beautifully sculpted body.

When it comes to losing weight and getting in shape, mental readiness is everything. Sometimes conditions are good; sometimes they are not. You will be more successful if the time is right and you are prepared and emotionally ready.

Sometimes life is rosy, but sometimes it is complicated. You might be dealing with job pressures, financial stress, relationship problems—or even positive stresses like falling in love or getting a promotion. Complicated times like these are difficult points at which to begin a program. They may distract you, can sap your energy, and can make your environment less than supportive. Think about how your life events will influence your chances for success.

This issue of readiness should not be interpreted as deciding whether it will ever be a good time to lose weight. It is more a question of whether now is the right time. If the answer is no, then it is time to start changing things so the right time will not be too far off. The first step in changing eating behavior is to understand the conditions that influence your eating habits.

If you know the conditions are right, congratulations! You are ready to begin.

I want so much for you to reach your goal and feel wonderful about your looks and your life. All of this is possible—and more, if you set yourself up to succeed. To assure that you achieve your desires, there are a few final things you need to know.

First, as crazy as it sounds, you might want to postpone dieting for a few weeks and focus on becoming more active. Why do I say this? One of the reasons you may have struggled with your weight up to now is inactivity. As bad as it is to be overweight, it may be just as bad to be inactive. In fact, some health authorities believe it is worse. The road to permanent weight loss will be so much smoother if you increase your physical activity.

Many people I know prepare by just starting Zumba first. Several sessions a week of Zumba will melt the weight off anybody. My assistant at Zumba Fitness, Vickie Zagarra, is a good example. Vickie, who is also the model in the dance and exercise photos in this book, has melted away sixty pounds. Her weight loss started when she began Zumba classes. Within a couple of weeks, before she had even considered dieting, the first ten pounds had vanished. Then something changed in her head. Vickie felt so good about herself that she did not want to put unhealthy food in her body anymore. Vickie was craving healthy foods, so she started eating more nutritiously. Her new way of eating came to her practically without effort. When you start feeling better about yourself through Zumba, you will be more mentally prepared to start the Zumba Diet.

Second, when you are ready to change your eating habits, prepare your social environment. Tell your family, friends, coworkers, and others in your social circle about your plans and ask them to support you. I do not mean, however, asking people you know to act like the "food police," watching your every move to make sure you stick to your diet. That does not work for most people and often fosters rebellion. In reality, social support means the opposite. It is having your family and friends empower you to lose weight.

Who should you look to for support? The best support comes from family and friends, according to research. Of course, you want someone who is objective and nonjudgmental. If your mom has been nagging you about your extra pounds, rule her out as a candidate and find someone less emotionally invested. For people who can help you eat right and exercise, some of the most inspiring supporters will be those who have been there and done that. Knowing that someone else knows what you are going through is psychologically a boost, especially on the low days. There might be people you know through Zumba who can make a huge difference.

Make a list of at least three friends or family members you could ask to help you toward your goal. Make regular contact—exercise or cook together, share recipes and/or discuss your progress. If you have started and stopped diet or exercise plans with people in the past, do not turn to them this time; seek out others. Push yourself to meet new people, perhaps at the gym or in Zumba.

If none of your friends is interested in eating well, find some who are. Internet support groups are great for this. You may end up becoming the inspiration for your old friends.

Third, make sure you have the right foods available. Most overeating is due to poor planning. Not even the best diet in the world can help you if your refrigerator is full of nothing but cake! So make sure you have lots of good food available at all times. Clear your house of foods you have a history of abusing—cookies, chips, chocolate, peanuts, ice cream—whatever is your trigger. It is amazing what a well-stocked refrigerator full of delicious, prepared food does for preventing that desire to eat junk food. Most of your cravings and uncontrolled overeating will be conquered when you feed your body what it needs regularly during the day and you have the food at your fingertips when you need it. We are more likely to eat whatever is in our environment. If you surround yourself with delicious, healthy, wholesome foods, that is what you will end up eating.

Try to make things easy on yourself, too. Get in the habit of preparing bulk meals, preferably on weekends when you have some leisure time. For example, whip up a big batch of grains once or twice a week, then simply add fresh veggies and light proteins. To further cut down on prep time, use precut chicken and shelled, deveined shrimp, along with prechopped frozen or fresh onions, bell peppers, other veggies, and garlic.

The idea is to fix quick and easy dinners so that you always have something in the freezer or refrigerator that is ready to serve on a moment's notice and purchase only what is on your shopping list at the market (being open, of course, to varying your selection of produce based on what is in season).

Finally, think fun, not deprivation. Starting a weight-loss plan does not mean subjecting yourself to a diet of rabbit food. The foods on the Zumba Diet are delicious and good for you, and you will lose weight gradually without feeling deprived. Make enjoying beautiful, delicious, and healthy foods your mission. Scan supermarket shelves for the sweetest exotic fruit, the juiciest tomatoes of the season, and the most fragrant herbs. Eat well, reward yourself with a pretty table setting, and you will stay positive and focused on success.

THE EXCITING FIRST STEP TO A BETTER SHAPE

You can begin the Zumba Diet with a kick-start plan to take pounds off quickly. This is called the Zumba 5-Day Express Diet. It is designed to give you a little edge. If you stick to it faithfully, you could find yourself lighter by up to nine pounds after five days. Isn't that incredible? Many people find that starting off with a few days of major calorie cutting and losing a lot of weight initially actually provides an incentive to stick with a more moderate weight-loss plan. This five-day diet can flip a switch in the way you behave, and often in how you feel and think. You should feel lighter and more energized, for example. It may also make you realize that you do not need as much food as you have been eating.

Of course, a little of your weight loss on the Zumba 5-Day Express Diet is generally water weight, but seeing that drop on the scale can definitely motivate you to keep going. You can keep losing pounds after the first five days if you then switch to a well-balanced low-fat, modified-carb diet that you can stick with over time—which is what the Zumba Diet offers. The several pounds you shed after five days gives you the morale boost to help you continue with the Zumba Diet—and ultimately lose fifteen to twenty pounds over two months.

If your weight ever reaches a plateau—in other words, you are stalled in dropping off pounds—you can use the Zumba 5-Day Express Diet again to break the plateau. It is a great tool to keep the numbers on your scale going down.

So if you are ready, let's get a jump on all this by starting the Zumba 5-Day Express Diet.

Chapter 9

THE ZUMBA 5-DAY EXPRESS DIET

Sometimes we need to see real progress at the start of a diet to motivate us through the day-in, day-out sensible, healthy regimen of keeping portions down; curbing intake of fatty, sugary, and salty foods; and staying active. Having worked as a fitness instructor and personal trainer for almost twenty years, I have talked to people about diet countless times. And while I know that slow, steady weight loss is the best way to lose pounds and keep them off, I also know that sometimes you need a little kick-start that only a few days of a serious calorie-cutback provides.

Even research supports what I am saying. From a psychological perspective, fast weight loss early on can predict longer-term success. So with the Zumba 5-Day Express Diet, you will give your weight loss a jump-start and help keep yourself going.

Mark my words: This part of the diet is an easy way to shed pounds rapidly, over five days, and experience a quick drop in weight that will give you a powerful mental boost.

Is it really possible to shed pounds swiftly yet safely? Yes. As long as your diet does not last longer than five days, you do not have to sacrifice your nutritional needs. You will not be faint with hunger, and five days is not that long. This diet is something anyone can do. Afterward, you can look forward to a more liberal way of eating—and keep losing weight.

Depending on your weight when you start out, you can expect to lose up to five pounds by following this high-nutrient plan. Although individual results vary, *we have seen people lose as many as nine pounds in five days!*

If your diet has been very salty up to this point, you will drop weight even faster, because you will be eliminating sodium, the mineral found in table salt. Salt contains no calories, so it does not make you fatter. But if you eat a lot of salt, you retain fluid, and you will look heavier. And you can be heavier on the scale (by three to five pounds) for as long as three days when there is too much sodium in your diet.

After beginning the Zumba 5-Day Express Diet, some of your loss will be water, and that is awesome, because water is weight, too. Never dismiss those extra pounds as only "water weight"; this is a self-defeating attitude. Shedding water weight is healthy. Cosmetically, water weight can hide fat loss and be particularly frustrating. Healthwise, fluid retention can put a strain on the heart because of the extra volume of blood it is required to pump.

Once all of that extra fluid has departed, so will your bloat and puffiness. You will start looking visibly thinner in three or four days. And chances are you will feel much lighter and, I hope, be motivated to watch what you eat in the long run.

You will feel so delighted by the rapid loss of a few pounds that you will decide to keep on going on the full Zumba Diet. So if you start the Zumba 5-Day Express Diet on Monday, by the weekend you could be a few pounds lighter, and that little black number hiding in your closet could get an airing at last!

In a nutshell, the Zumba 5-Day Express Diet is based on burning fat, controlling your hunger, reducing bloat, and giving you a psychological boost from dropping pounds quickly. You will love the way you look and feel after only five days, and you will be inspired to start the Zumba Diet.

Don't worry, the Zumba 5-Day Express Diet is not a fast. Fasts are unhealthy, and can leave you feeling sick and weak. They can backfire on you and may spur a massive eating binge after a couple of days.

The Zumba 5-Day Express Diet is not difficult. It is easy to follow. There are no feelings of deprivation or cravings. You will not feel like anything is being taken away from you—only unwanted pounds and inches. You can stick to it when you travel, when you go out to restaurants, or when you entertain. And you will feel energized while you are on it, because you are eating such wholesome, nutrient-rich food. This five-day eating plan is fast, and it will work for you.

So, are you ready to kick your weight loss into high gear?

Are you ready to shed pounds this week?

Are you ready to look fabulous and feel fit?

Without further ado, let's move on to the Zumba 5-Day Express Diet.

GENERAL INSTRUCTIONS

You will be reducing your food intake slightly for five days by following a specific five-day menu plan. When your body senses this reduction, it taps into, and burns, body fat for energy. Instead of focusing on portion control or on counting calories, the five-day plan emphasizes the type of food you should eat for weight loss, energy, and health. This plan combines a healthful mix of nutrients, with most of the calories coming from vegetables, fruits, proteins, and some fat. You will be including a number of the bodyshaping foods discussed in the previous chapter—foods that enhance the fat-burning process and help you improve your shape. All the foods on the diet are ordinary foods, available in all supermarkets. There is a wide choice to suit all tastes.

To ensure that the weight comes off, steadily and healthfully, please follow these instructions:

1. Eat exactly what is listed.

In other words, do not substitute. This also means not skipping meals. If your body gets used to not eating for long stretches, it will adapt by conserving energy and reducing the number of calories it burns. Your metabolism will go into starvation mode, and your body will burn up fewer calories.

The menus are preplanned for you. Knowing what is to be eaten prevents having to make food decisions when you are vulnerable. If you slip, return to healthy, moderate eating the next day. Do not let a single mistake with a load of calories undermine what you are doing.

2. Do not skip breakfast.

Breakfast is vital. When you sleep your body uses less energy so it can focus on repairing damage. By the time you wake up, your body is in full-on conservation mode and burning calories very slowly. If you do not give it food within an hour of waking, it does not realize you are up and continues to burn fat more slowly for the rest of the day.

3. Eat until you are satisfied, not stuffed.

Where no portion is indicated, you can eat as much as you like, but never overload your stomach. When you feel full, *stop*! Listen to your appetite and adjust your eating accordingly.

4. Enjoy between-meal snacks.

If you feel hungry at any time, make sure you are drinking enough water. Physiologically, thirst often masquerades as hunger. You need at least eight cups of pure water daily, or more. For snacks, have on hand lots of vegetables, which will nip hunger pangs in the bud. These include raw cauliflower, broccoli, and baby carrots.

5. Take a multivitamin and mineral supplement.

With any diet, it is a good idea to have extra nutritional insurance. Select a supplement that supplies about 100 percent of all the nutrients listed on the label. Check with your doctor prior to taking supplements.

6. Do not stay on the diet more than five days at a time.

The five-day diet is designed to give you a positive jump-start and make you feel confident about what your body can accomplish. At the end of five days, you will be physically and mentally ready to start the more liberal Zumba Diet. The five-day diet is a tool to help you speed up your weight loss, but is not meant as a long-term plan.

7. Use the Zumba 5-Day Express Diet as a tool.

You can use the Zumba 5-Day Express Diet to break a frustrating weight-loss plateau or keep weight fluctuations to a minimum, get back on track if you have overindulged, fit into a new size by the weekend, and lose those stubborn last five pounds. The diet is a tool you can use to get the results you want.

Here is something else very cool: researchers have discovered that phasing a low-calorie diet (like the Zumba 5-Day Express Diet) in and out of regular, more moderate dieting burns more pure fat than if you just stick to weeks and weeks of continuous, moderate dieting. It is believed that the caloric ups and downs can boost your metabolism to burn fat.

So you might consider phasing in the Zumba 5-Day Express Diet in the following manner:

Five-day diet—1 month of the Zumba Diet—five-day diet—1 month of the Zumba Diet—five-day diet—and so forth.

Caution: People with chronic conditions such as diabetes, low or high blood sugar, high blood pressure, or cardiac arrhythmia should never drop their calorie counts drastically. Also, beware that dramatic changes in diet can affect the dosage of some prescription medicines you may be taking. Again, check with your doctor before starting any diet.

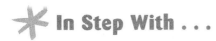 **In Step With . . .**

Margarita Hernandez Kohler, Memphis, Tennessee

Margarita, age forty, had been overweight for more than ten years. After each pregnancy—she has two daughters—Margarita put on pounds and could not take them off. By 2004, she weighed in at 200 pounds, only to gain twenty more over the next two years. She was down, but not out. Margarita was determined to make a change in her life.

"I started to walk, since that was the only thing I could do," she says. "I cut out all junk and fast food, such as pizza, hamburgers, fries, chips, sodas, and cookies."

Before long, Margarita was feeling strong enough to join a dance fitness class at a local sports club. At first she was embarrassed, afraid people would snicker behind her back. She imagined they were calling her a "dancing bear."

The class became a Zumba class, and at the time nobody knew what that was. But as soon as Margarita, who was born in Mexico, discovered that it was a Latin rhythm class, she never missed a session.

After becoming a healthier eater and working out six to seven days a week, Margarita lost seventy-five pounds. It was a rebirth for her. "The fact that I can move again—and dance—makes me cry. Zumba gave me back my life."

ARE YOU READY? WHAT TO DO THE DAY BEFORE

There is something important I suggest you do now: Head to the supermarket and pick up all the foods you will need for the next five days. That way, you will have the right food in stock. (See the shopping list on the next page.)

There is one other thing I would like you to do: Weigh yourself on the morning of day one, and record your weight in a notebook.

Now you are ready—to take off pounds and forge a wonderfully healthy new way of eating and exercising!

SHOPPING LIST FOR THE ZUMBA 5-DAY EXPRESS DIET

Ready to hit the supermarket? Here's a shopping list—and when you're in the store, resist the temptation to buy anything else.

STAPLES	VEGETABLES	FRUIT	RESISTANT STARCHES
Balsamic vinegar	1 bag spinach leaves	2 to 3 grapefruits, or other citrus fruits	1 box high-fiber cereal (All-Bran, All-Bran Bran Buds, Fiber One, etc.)
Cocktail sauce	3 bags mixed greens	½ pint berries (any variety), or 1 or 2 bags of frozen unsweetened berries	
Cider vinegar	1 cucumber		
Crushed red pepper	1 onion		1 loaf high-fiber whole-wheat bread
Fat-free mayonnaise	2 tomatoes		
Ground black pepper	Carton of cherry or grape tomatoes	2 or 3 small apples	1 container oatmeal or Cream of Wheat
Ground cumin		1 or 2 peaches or nectarines	
Hot pepper sauce	1 package of alfalfa sprouts		1 box uncooked brown rice
Mustard	1 to 2 green peppers		

<table>
<tr><td>No-sugar ketchup</td><td>1 small bag of baby carrots</td><td colspan="2" align="center">MEAT, FISH, AND POULTRY</td><td align="center">DAIRY</td></tr>
</table>

STAPLES	VEGETABLES	MEAT, FISH, AND POULTRY	DAIRY
No-sugar ketchup	1 small bag of baby carrots		
Salad spritzer		1 package skinless, boneless chicken breasts or chicken thighs	1 container fat-free plain yogurt
Vegetable oil cooking spray	Frozen or fresh veggies: asparagus, Brussels sprouts, broccoli, cauliflower, green beans, summer squash, zucchini, or other vegetable on list		1 carton fat-free cottage cheese
1 jar mild fat-free salsa		1 piece of fish or large portion of shellfish	1 dozen large eggs
Coffee		1 steak	1 package crumbled fat-free feta cheese
Green tea		1 skinless boneless turkey breast	1 quart skim milk or non-dairy milk
	1 bunch celery	1 package low-fat, low-sodium deli chicken slices	
	1 bunch basil		**OTHER ITEMS**
	1 bunch green onions	1 or 2 3-ounce cans tuna, water packed	1 can (10¾ ounces) condensed vegetable soup, low fat, low sodium

FIVE POUNDS (OR MORE) LIGHTER IN FIVE DAYS

Now for the diet. Keep this in mind as you get ready to start: This diet works when you work with it. If you feel like you are not losing weight, review the instructions on pages 170–171. Any deviation could throw things out of whack. Followed to the letter, the Zumba 5-Day Express Diet is your chance to start feeling lighter right away and tap into healthful living for the rest of your life.

BREAKFAST

For breakfast each day, you have two choices. Enjoy breakfast #1 or #2 each day, or alternate between them.

Breakfast #1

1 slice high-fiber toast, no spread added (*Note:* "High-fiber" refers to bread that contains 3 grams of fiber or more per slice.)

1 poached, hard-boiled, soft-boiled, or scrambled egg (prepared with vegetable cooking spray), or 1 serving egg substitute

1 serving of fresh fruit: ½ grapefruit, 1 small (3-inch diameter) orange, 1 small apple (3-inch diameter), 1 peach or nectarine, or 1 cup fresh berries (strawberries, blueberries, raspberries, or blackberries)

Coffee/tea (no sugar, no cream or milk, no honey)

Breakfast #2

1 cup high-fiber cold cereal (All-Bran, All-Bran Bran Buds, or Fiber One) or ½ cup cooked whole-grain cereal (oat bran, oatmeal, Cream of Wheat, or quinoa)

1 cup skim milk, soy milk, almond milk, or rice milk; or fat-free yogurt

1 serving of fresh fruit: ½ grapefruit, 1 small (3-inch diameter) orange, 1 small apple (3-inch diameter), 1 peach or nectarine, or 1 cup fresh berries (strawberries, blueberries, raspberries, or blackberries)

Coffee/green tea (no sugar, no cream or milk, no honey)

DAY ONE

Lunch

Soup and salad lunch: 1 soup bowl of fat-free, low-sodium vegetable soup (or our Garden Vegetable Soup recipe on page 249.)

1 plate of mixed salad greens and vegetables, any greens and salad vegetables, as you wish. A mixed salad can include lettuces, cucumber, onion, tomatoes, grated carrot, beetroot, celery, peppers, radish, bean sprouts, served with salad spritzer. A salad spritzer, which you can find near the salad dressings in the grocery store, is an excellent way to reduce fat and calories. Instead of pouring salad dressing onto your salad, you spray it on. Spritzers spray one calorie's worth of dressing at a time.

Coffee/green tea/water

Dinner

Roasted or baked chicken thighs or breasts (skin and visible fat removed before cooking). You can cook these with a little vegetable cooking spray.

Plenty of steamed Brussels sprouts, broccoli, cauliflower, or green beans—but no oil or fat should be added.

1 serving of fresh fruit: ½ grapefruit, 1 small (3-inch diameter) orange, 1 small apple (3-inch diameter), 1 peach or nectarine, or 1 cup fresh berries (strawberries, blueberries, raspberries, or blackberries)

Coffee/green tea/water

DAY TWO

Lunch

Large spinach salad: Fresh spinach torn into large pieces; low-fat feta cheese, crumbled; sliced mushrooms, sliced thin; thinly sliced red onion; cherry or grape tomatoes; served with salad spritzer

Coffee/green tea/water

Dinner

Baked fish or steamed shellfish, served with cocktail sauce

½ cup cooked brown rice

Plenty of steamed vegetables: summer squash, green beans, spinach, zucchini, broccoli, etc. (no oil or fat added)

Green tea/water

DAY THREE

Lunch

Chicken salad sandwich: 2 slices high-fiber bread, sliced fat-free smoked deli-style chicken, 1 tablespoon Dijon mustard, and lettuce

Sliced tomato salad: tomato slices, onion slices, and fresh basil (2 leaves), served with salad spritzer

Green tea/water

Dinner

Baked or broiled pork chops (2)—a little vegetable cooking spray can be used

Plenty of steamed vegetables: summer squash, green beans, spinach, zucchini, broccoli, etc. (no oil or fat added)

1 serving of fresh fruit: ½ grapefruit, 1 small (3-inch diameter) orange, 1 small apple (3-inch diameter), 1 peach or nectarine, or 1 cup fresh berries (strawberries, blueberries, raspberries, or blackberries)

Green tea/water

DAY FOUR

Lunch

Tuna-stuffed tomato: Partially slice 1 large tomato into quarters; stuff with tuna packed in water mixed with 2 tablespoons chopped celery, 1 tablespoons diced scallions, and 1 tablespoon fat-free mayonnaise

Green tea/water

Dinner

Roasted turkey breast (a little bit of vegetable cooking spray may be used for cooking)

½ cup cooked brown rice

Plenty of steamed vegetables: summer squash, green beans, spinach, zucchini, broccoli, etc. (no oil or fat added)

DAY FIVE

Lunch

Fruit salad: ½ cup fat-free cottage cheese or ½ cup fat-free yogurt served with orange segments, 1 cup fresh berries, and a sliced apple or peach, all on a bed of lettuce

Green tea/water

Dinner

Grilled or broiled steak, all visible fat removed before cooking; any cut of steak you wish: sirloin, rib-eye, porterhouse, eye of the round, etc.

Plenty of steamed Brussels sprouts, broccoli, cauliflower, or green beans (no oil or fat added)

1 plate of mixed salad greens and vegetables, any greens and salad vegetables, as you wish. A mixed salad can include lettuces, cucumber, onion, tomatoes, grated carrot, beetroot, celery, peppers, radish, bean sprouts, served with salad spritzer.

Green tea/water

Eating Out on the Five-Day Diet

It is probably a good idea to avoid restaurants during the five days you are following this diet. Your weight loss will be more satisfying if you prepare the meals yourself. However, if you do go out to eat, restaurants do not have to be your downfall! If you order carefully, choosing baked, broiled, or grilled chicken or fish, along with vegetables, you will do well on the Zumba 5-Day Express Diet. You can eat out and enjoy it. Here's how:

* Try to select restaurants where ordering will not be a challenge. It is tough to get what you want at a French or an Italian restaurant, for example. Steak-and-seafood-type restaurants are your best bet.

✳ Rather than an alcoholic drink for dinner, order a club soda with a lime or lemon. Sip it and you will find that it fills you up, taking the edge off your hunger. Alcohol, on the other hand, lowers your inhibitions, so you're more apt to have another drink (or two) and mow through appetizers even before the main course.

✳ Ask the waitperson not to bring the bread basket.

✳ Order a green salad with your meal, without the dressing. Then pull out your salad spritzer to flavor your salad.

✳ Ask how entrées are prepared (grilled is usually better than fried, for instance), order sauces on the side, and skip toppings like cheese to keep yourself on track. Also, ask that your entrées, like chicken, fish, or meat, as well as vegetables, be prepared without oil, butter, or margarine. (You will find more eating-out tips on pages 235–239.)

Zumba and the Five-Day Diet

Continue your Zumba schedule while following the five-day diet. For optimum fueling, consider doing Zumba an hour after you have eaten a meal. Zumba burns a lot of calories while you are doing it, and your metabolism continues to burn fat faster for some time afterward since it is aerobic exercise. But Zumba also includes strength-training components to help you develop and maintain lean muscle. The best way to fire up your metabolism is to increase your lean tissue through this type of exercise, because muscle burns nine times more calories than fat. Remember, gain muscle and you will burn fat even when you are asleep, and your body will look leaner. You do not have to pump iron, as you can use your own body weight as resistance with Zumba moves like lunges, squats, crunches, and other sculpting moves.

What to Do after the Five Days Are Up

The first thing I want you to do is weigh yourself on the morning of the sixth day. Try on the outfit that was snug a week ago, and note the difference in how it fits. If you have done everything to the letter, you should be at least several pounds lighter. Then congratulate yourself!

After you come off the diet, your stomach should feel smaller, and your body more averse to junk foods. Shedding extra pounds should bring you a confidence boost, and you will love your trimmer figure and clearer eyes and skin. Another benefit will be your increased energy levels.

At the end of the first five days—with a few pounds less under your belt—you may be tempted to take your weight loss and run—straight to the nearest ice cream sundae. But do not do that! To stay on track and lose more weight, follow the Zumba Diet. Detailed instructions begin in the next chapter.

The Zumba 5-Day Diet is just the beginning. It gives you a positive, affirming jump-start, and the confidence, I hope, to continue your great progress.

Isn't it fun to look good, be full of energy, and to fall in love with yourself again?

Chapter 10
THE ZUMBA DIET

Now let's get into the specifics of the Zumba Diet. The best part (besides all the fat you will lose) is that it emphasizes real food, and lots of it, to help you get more fit. The high-quality food selections in this plan are used by the body to develop muscle, burn off fat, enhance your shape, and energize you. There are five groups of food—light proteins, resistant starches, high-volume vegetables, fruits, and healthy fats—that will accomplish this.

Let me explain these five food groups in more detail.

LIGHT PROTEINS

I am sure you would turn up your nose at some of the traditional proteins we eat at a Colombian meal. Let me put it this way: In Colombia, we believe in using every bit of a chicken, pig, or cow for food and not wasting an ounce! But for losing weight and reshaping your body, you have to be more picky than that—which brings me to the issue of protein.

You want protein because it provides building blocks called amino acids to make your lean muscle tissue develop. Protein not only adds to your muscle, which is key in boosting the metabolism, but it actually increases your metabolism more directly. The body burns more calories processing protein than it burns to process carbs or fat, in a reaction known as thermogenesis. This reaction explains why higher-protein diets result in greater fat loss than lower-protein diets, even when both diets contain the same number of calories. Protein also stimulates fat-burning in the abdominal region of the body. What's more, protein is slow to digest, which means you feel fuller longer.

Light protein includes all your lean meats, poultry, fish, shellfish, soy protein, and low-fat dairy products.

Daily Allotment: Eat a serving of light protein for breakfast, lunch, and dinner. You can also enjoy smaller portions of light protein for snacks.

Here is a complete list of light proteins:

Meats and Poultry

Beef (lean cuts only): Bottom round, eye of the round, round tip (sirloin tip), tenderloin, top loin (strip loin), top round, top sirloin, lean ground meat (*Note*: Be moderate with red meat. If you like red meat, enjoy it a few times a week, not every day.)

Chicken breast, skin removed

Chicken thighs, skin removed

Cornish game hen, skin removed

Eggs*

Lamb

Lunch meats—reduced fat or nonfat

Pork chops, lean

Turkey breast, skin removed

Turkey, ground, lean

Turkey, reduced-fat products (sausage, bacon, luncheon meat, etc.)

Veal

† People with high cholesterol or who have been told by their doctors to reduce cholesterol for any reason should eat no more than three eggs a week.

Prep Tips: Meat and poultry can be broiled, grilled, baked, roasted, microwaved, or sautéed with nonstick vegetable spray. Marinating these foods in fat-free salad dressings can help add extra flavor without extra calories. All meat should be very lean; remove all visible fat before eating. Remove skin and fat from poultry before eating. The skin is loaded with calories. In a whole chicken, the meat contains about 800 calories, while the skin has a whopping 2,000 calories!

Be careful not to undercook meat, poultry, or fish, however. Undercooking increases the risk that illness-causing bacteria will form on the food. With meat, for example, cook it to the medium rare or medium stage to be on the safe side. Chicken and fish should be fully cooked.

Going Organic: You can buy "natural beef" that has been raised without chemicals. Instead of using hormones to promote growth, ranchers allow the animals more time to graze, and veterinarians treat disease with less conventional means rather than with antibiotics. Many scientists are concerned about the antibiotics being given to most farm animals. Many are the same antibiotics humans rely on, and overuse of these drugs has already enabled bacteria to develop resistance to them, making them less effective in fighting infection. Thus organic meats may offer some health benefits, although they are not necessary for losing weight. When shopping for organic foods, always look for the USDA seal on any kind of packaged food. For meat and dairy, this seal ensures you are getting antibiotic- and hormone-free products.

Free-Range Poultry: "Free range" means chicken and turkeys are not raised in coops or given antibiotics or hormones to boost growth. Although more expensive than conventionally raised poultry, free-range birds are often leaner and thus lower in fat because they are not as sedentary.

Fish and Shellfish

Bass	Orange roughy
Bluefish	Oysters
Catfish	Perch
Clams	Pollock
Cod	Red snapper
Crabmeat	Salmon, canned and drained, or fresh*
Flounder	Sardines, packed in water, mustard, or
Grouper	tomato sauce*
Haddock	Scallops
Halibut*	Shark
Herring*	Shrimp
Lobster	Sole
Mackerel*	Swordfish
Monkfish	Tilapia
Mussels	Trout
	Tuna (fresh or low-sodium canned)*

*Omega-3 Fish: Fish marked with an asterisk are high in omega-3 fats, a type of polyunsaturated fatty acid found in salmon, sardines, mackerel, halibut, and albacore tuna (canned or fresh). Omega-3 fats are good for the body, heart, and brain. The American Heart Association recommends eating omega-3-rich fatty fish two times per week.

Prep Tip: You can sauté, bake, grill, microwave, or poach fish. It is fully cooked when it flakes easily with a fork. Do not fry your fish. Frying in oil adds lots of fat and calories and defeats the purpose of eating fish. Use water, bouillon, or vegetable cooking spray instead.

Farm-Raised versus Wild: Farm fish, particularly salmon, are frequently fed smaller fish that are ground up and made into pellets. This feeding practice boosts their risk of accumulated contaminants, compared with wild-caught fish. If this is a concern, you do not have to eliminate all farm-raised fish. Several farmed species pose less risk, including mussels, trout, catfish, and clams.

Seafood and Mercury: If you are worried about reports that environmental contaminants exist in certain species of seafood, vary the types of fish you eat. Atlantic herring, wild sockeye salmon, and Atlantic cod are among the fish with the lowest mercury levels. Larger species of fish, like king mackerel, tilefish, shark, and swordfish, contain higher levels. Never eat the skin of fish, either. It is a main storage area for toxins.

Low-Fat Dairy

Fat-free plain yogurt

Fat-free, sugar-free, fruit-flavored yogurt

Low-fat cottage cheese

Cheeses

Skim milk

Nondairy choices such as: soy milk, almond milk, or rice milk

Prep tip: These foods are delicious on their own, or they can be used in recipes to replace cream, full-fat cheeses, or other higher-fat dairy items.

Soy Protein

Edamame (boiled and sometimes salted soybeans in the pod or without the pod)

Soybeans

Soy burgers or hot dogs

Soy milk, calcium fortified

Tempeh

Textured vegetable protein

Tofu

Using Soy: Soy protein is a great health food. It helps in weight control, heart health, and overall well-being. Soy is easy to add to your diet. Some suggestions: Use soy milk on your cereal and blended into smoothies. Try soy burgers in place of hamburgers. Use textured soy protein in recipes calling for ground beef. Snack on soy-based energy bars, rather than on candy bars. Use tofu in Italian recipes like lasagna to replace all or part of the ricotta cheese. Tofu can also be blended into shakes and smoothies, plus used as a base for dips. *Caution:* Do not go overboard on soy foods. Too much soy in the diet may cause mineral deficiencies. If you like soy, enjoy it in moderation—a few servings a week.

RESISTANT STARCH AND OTHER HEALTHY STARCHES

In the city of Cali, where I grew up, our most traditional dish is a popular soup called *sancocho*. It is made mostly of hen, plantains, corn, and various seasonings, and is frequently eaten with banana slices. It sounds very high carb, and carbohydrates have certainly developed a bad name over the years. However, I learned that this soup is high in a healthful carbohydrate called "resistant starch."

Discovered by scientists in the early 1980s, resistant starch is a component of certain carbohydrates that "resists" digestion. In other words, it is not completely digested or absorbed in the small intestines as other foods are. Resistant starch thus never enters the bloodstream. That means it bypasses the fate of most carbs, which can get deposited as body fat if you eat more than you can burn off. Instead, resistant starch migrates to the large intestine, where it acts like fiber.

By eating a meal containing resistant starch, you can burn 20 to 25 percent more fat throughout the day. Scientists who study how resistant starch works in the body say that it actually changes the order in which the body burns food. Usually carbohydrates are used first, but resistant starch seems to move fat to the top of the list to be burned for energy before it has a chance to be stored.

Resistant Starches

Carbohydrates containing resistant starch are what we push in the Zumba Diet. The top sources of resistant starch include:

Beans (kidney, pinto, black, garbanzo beans, and so forth)

Bananas (slightly green)

Yams

Sweet potatoes

Potatoes

Barley

Brown rice

Corn, including low-fat creamed corn

We will also focus on other healthy carbohydrates such as whole-grain cereals, high-fiber cereals, whole-grain breads, whole-grain pastas, starchy vegetables like winter squash, and many more. All carbohydrates provide the basic energy for your body. In their most natural state (unrefined), carbohydrates also supply fiber. Because fibrous foods provide bulk, you feel full while eating a meal, so you are less tempted to overeat. High-fiber foods also take longer to chew, so your meals last longer. That is a plus, since it takes about twenty minutes after starting a meal for your body to send signals that it is full. And, when eaten with other nutrients like protein, fiber slows the rate of digestion, too, curbing your appetite between meals. As a bodyshaping food, fiber in ample amounts (at least twenty-six grams daily) in your diet helps scale down your thighs, according to research.

Daily Allotment: Eat three servings a day of recommended starches.

Here is a complete list of starches:

Breads

Cracked wheat	Pumpernickel
High-fiber bread	Raisin
Mixed grain	Rye, light or dark
Oatmeal	Whole wheat
Pita, whole wheat	Tortillas, corn or low-carb flour

Cold Cereals

All-Bran	Raisin Bran
All-Bran Extra Fiber	Shredded Wheat
All-Bran Bran Buds	Wheat bran (use 1–2 tablespoons sprinkled on other cereals)
Multi-Bran Chex	
Fiber One	Wheat germ (use 1–2 tablespoons sprinkled on other cereals)

Cooked Cereals

Corn grits	Oat bran
Cream of Wheat	Oatmeal

Grain Products

Amaranth	Couscous
Barley, pearl	Millet
Bulgur wheat	Quinoa

Rice and Pasta

Spinach pasta	Brown rice
Whole-wheat pasta	Wild rice

Starchy Vegetables

Beets	Pumpkin
Peas	Squash, winter (acorn, butternut, Hubbard, etc.)

Prep Tip: Store grains in a dark, dry spot in tightly sealed containers. If you live in a humid climate, you can store grains safely in the refrigerator for up to a year. Never rinse rice or other grains prior to cooking. Rinsing washes away nutrients and devitalizes the grain. With the exception of cold high-fiber cereals, starches can be boiled, steamed, or microwaved—and prepared without added fat, sugar, or salt.

HIGH-VOLUME VEGETABLES

High-volume vegetables are composed primarily of water, vitamins, minerals, and fiber. They are low in calories and contain no fat or added sugar. You can eat a lot of them, feel full, and still lose weight.

High-volume vegetables include broccoli, Brussels sprouts, cauliflower, cabbage, carrots, onions, tomatoes, squash, and green, leafy vegetables such as lettuce and spinach. You cannot go wrong loading up on vegetables. Researchers have learned that people who eat the widest variety of vegetables have the least body fat. This research is a wonderful testimony to the power of vegetables in maintaining a healthy weight.

Daily Allotment: You can enjoy vegetables at lunch and dinner—and eat them to your heart's content. Try to vary your selection of vegetables from day to day to get the most from these wonderful foods.

High-Volume Vegetables

Alfalfa sprouts	Celery
Artichokes	Collard greens
Arugula	Cucumber
Asparagus	Dandelion greens
Beet greens	Eggplant
Bok choy	Endive
Broccoli	Garlic
Brussels sprouts	Green beans
Cabbage	Jicama
Cauliflower	Kale

Kohlrabi	Rutabaga
Leeks	Scallions
Lettuce, all varieties	Spinach
Mushrooms	Summer squash, all varieties
Mustard greens	Swiss chard
Okra	Tomatoes
Onions	Turnip greens
Parsley	Turnips
Parsnips	Watercress
Pea pods	Yellow (wax) beans
Peppers, all varieties	Zucchini
Radishes	

Soups*

Bean soup	Vegetable soup
Lentil soup	Vegetarian chili

* Recommended soups are those low in fat and sodium.

Prep Tips: There is a lot you can do to get the most nutrition from vegetables. Some suggestions:

* Look for fresh produce that is crisp and not wilted. Fresh equates with nutritious.

* When purchasing a salad mix, look for a colorful medley of greens in the bag. The more color, the more nutrients in the salad.

✳ Go for darker shades of green when purchasing lettuce. Dark-leafed vegetables like romaine lettuce are richer in many vitamins than are lighter green varieties of lettuce such as iceberg. Similarly, buy certain vegetables, such as onions and sweet peppers, in all their various colors, for a greater array of nutrients.

✳ When buying from a salad bar, avoid vegetables that look brown or slimy. These indicate that the produce has been stored at improper temperatures and may thus be nutritionally empty.

✳ Buy a variety of produce. The greater the variety of foods you eat, the more health-building nutrients you get in your diet.

✳ Wash fresh produce to remove surface dirt and bacteria, but do not soak it. With soaking, nutrients leach out into the water.

✳ Cook foods for the shortest amount of time possible. Use your microwave for quick cooking and for reheating leftovers. Quick-cooking methods, at high temperatures with the least exposure to water, preserve the greatest amount of nutrients. By contrast, vitamins in vegetables are easily destroyed with prolonged exposure to heat, water, and air. Other good quick-cooking methods include steaming, stir-frying, and grilling.

✳ Cook vegetables using a steam basket that fits into a saucepan. Fill the saucepan with an inch or two of water. Place vegetables in the basket and cover the saucepan with a tight-fitting lid. Steam vegetables for a few minutes—until tender but still crisp in order to preserve more nutrients.

✳ In lieu of a steam basket, fill the saucepan with an inch or less of water. Add vegetables so that they are piled above the water line. Cook for a just few minutes. The point is to reduce contact with water. Water dissolves water-soluble vitamins, such as vitamin C and the B vitamins.

✳ Try some of the frozen packaged vegetables marketed as "steamers." You simply pop the bag into the microwave for several minutes and the veggies steam right in the bag. This is an ultra-convenient, quick way to enjoy steamed vegetables.

✳ Cook vegetables with their skins on; this helps lock in nutrients. Consider mashing red potatoes with their skins on for greater nutritional value.

✳ Choose from fresh, frozen, and canned vegetables, though canned veggies are usually higher in salt. You can steam, boil, roast, or grill your vegetables, but do so without added fat or salt. Nonstick cooking spray may be used in moderation, however.

Going organic: Technically, the term "organic" does not describe how nutritious a food is. Rather, it means that the food has been produced, stored, processed, and packaged without the use of synthetic fertilizers, herbicides, fungicides, or pesticides. Organic foods may have higher nutritional value than conventional food, however, according to some research. The reason: Because they do not contain pesticides and fertilizers, plants boost their production of the phytochemicals (vitamins and antioxidants) that strengthen their resistance to bugs and weeds. Some studies have linked pesticides in our food to everything from headaches to cancer to birth defects.

FRUITS

Growing up in Colombia, I enjoyed many varieties of fruit virtually unknown outside the tropics, such as the zapote, lulo, curuba (banana passion fruit), mamoncillo, uchuva (gooseberry), feijoa, and sweet granadilla. You will also enjoy fruit on this plan, although not as exotic as these, but delicious nonetheless.

Fruit is highly nutritious, packed with vitamin C and other vitamins, fiber, and other health-building substances. Apples and pears are excellent sources of pectin, for example, a type of fiber that helps to reduce cholesterol levels. Dark-skinned berries such as blueberries, strawberries, raspberries, and blackberries have all been shown to contain powerful antioxidants called "bioflavonoids" that help protect the body's cells. Fruit also satisfies your cravings for sweets.

The best way to eat fruit is simply to eat it fresh. Ripe, sweet fruit in its prime makes a wonderful dessert, snack, or addition to any meal.

Daily Allotment: Eat two to three servings of fruit daily.

Fruit Choices

Apple, small	Melon
Apricot	Nectarine
Banana	Orange
Blackberries	Papaya
Blueberries	Peach
Cherries	Pear
Figs, fresh or dry	Pineapple
Grapefruit	Plum
Grapes	Prunes, stewed, unsweetened
Guava	Raspberries
Kiwi	Strawberries
Lemon	Tangelos
Lime	Tangerines
Mango	

Prep Tips: Nutrients in produce are very sensitive to exposure to heat, light, water, and oxygen. That being the case, you want to preserve the nutrient value of your food by following these important tips:

✳ When buying fresh fruits, be on the lookout for bruises on the fruit. Bruising initiates a chemical reaction that causes nutrient content to dwindle.

✳ Always select the brightest, most colorful fruits on the shelves. The brighter the color, the more vitamins and other nutrients the produce contains.

* Buy locally grown produce. It tends to be more nutrient rich because it comes picked right from the field to the produce stand, with less transit time in between. Nutrient loss occurs during the period between harvest and delivery at supermarkets.

* Berries are highly perishable. At the store, check for freshness by looking at the bottom of the box. Staining indicates that the fruit has been bruised or is overripe, meaning that it will spoil rapidly and that nutrient loss has already set in.

* Look for a bright red color when purchasing strawberries. Bright color signals exceptional nutritional quality. Avoid berries with too much whiteness at the base; they're less nutritious. Fruits such as cantaloupes and mangoes should feel somewhat soft to the touch.

* Avoid peeling, too. Nutrients and fiber are lost when produce is peeled.

HEALTHY FATS

Fats are as different from each other as an alley cat is from a tiger. Saturated fats (the bad fats) are found in animal fats, full-fat dairy products, margarine, palm oil, and coconut oil. These nasty fats are used widely in commercially baked products. Rates of bowel and prostate cancers, as well as coronary disease, increase in proportion to the amount of saturated fat in a person's diet. Polyunsaturated fats (these are sometimes called "the neutral fats") include many of the vegetable oils (safflower, corn, and soy) used in salad dressings. They are certainly better than saturated fats and reduce cholesterol, but they also reduce the good cholesterol (HDL) that take bad fats out of the body.

So what is left? The monounsaturated fats. These are the good fats that include olive oil, olives, nuts, fish, avocados, and canola oil. A diet of moderate monounsaturated fats helps reduce tummy fat and improves heart health. Fat also has an appetite-suppressing effect. That's because it is slow to digest and thus makes you feel full after you have eaten a meal.

Daily Allotment: Eat up to two servings daily of healthy fat. Serving sizes for different fats vary considerably, so they are listed next to the corresponding fat.

Healthy Fat Choices

Avocado (¼)	Peanut butter (2 tablespoons)
Almonds, raw or roasted without oil (14)	Sesame/sunflower seeds (2 tablespoons)
Brazil nuts (4)	Walnuts (8)
Canola oil (1 tablespoon)	Pine nuts (2 tablespoons)
Flaxseed oil (1 tablespoon)	Olive oil (1 tablespoon)
Hazelnuts (11)	Olives (20)

NUTRITIONAL BODYSHAPING

The Zumba Diet will help you burn overall fat, but if you have specific problem areas like a large tummy or big thighs, you will want to apply the principle of targeted dieting to your meal planning. To do that, figure out what you want to work on. A flatter belly? Thinner thighs? Or overall slimming? Then plan your meals around the bodyshaping foods that will help you manage those troublesome areas. For example:

For a Trimmer Tummy

✳ Stick to monounsaturated fats: nuts and seeds, avocados, peanut butter, olives, olive oil, canola oil, and flaxseed oil. This tip is based on recent research that shows that monounsaturated fatty acids actually can help reduce belly fat, including what medical experts call "visceral" fat, which is packed around your vital organs. Visceral fat has been linked to a variety of diseases, including diabetes, breast cancer, heart disease, and dementia. At the same time, avoid saturated fats such as butter, animal fat and cream, and hydrogenated (aka "trans") fats. These fats interfere with metabolism.

✳ Enjoy calcium-rich proteins such as yogurt, skim milk, and calcium-fortified soy milk. These foods help you lose weight and have been shown in research to shrink your belly. Suggested serving is two to three servings a day.

✳ Select whole grains as your starch choices for most meals. Researchers have found that whole grains reduce fat around the waistline. I am talking about stuff like oatmeal, brown rice, wild rice, barley, bulgur wheat, whole-wheat bread, and whole-wheat pasta.

For Thinner Thighs

The key here is to increase the fiber in your diet. In women, a high-fiber diet has been shown to reduce estrogen in the body. Estrogen is a hormone that, among other functions, directs fat to the thighs and hips. Scientists are not sure, but they think that by reducing estrogen naturally, with fiber, less fat gets deposited on the lower body.

The amount of fiber required to help reduced thigh circumference is at least twenty-six grams a day. It is generally recommended that adults get twenty-five to thirty-five grams of fiber a day anyway. Among the best choices are foods such as beans, peas, and lentils; rice, oats, barley, corn, and wheat bran; pears, apples, oranges, berries; carrots, potatoes, and squash; corn; seeds; nuts; whole-grain breads, cereals, and pasta; and green beans, broccoli, spinach, and tomatoes. The table below will help you identify various foods, along with their fiber content.

Another important point is to steer clear of fatty foods and foods high in sugar, especially if you are a woman. High-fat foods pack more calories and can more easily be stored as fat on the lower body.

Some experts believe that fatty foods and sugary foods contribute to cellulite, an accumulation of fat cells that are trapped in the protein (collagen and elastin) fibers of the skin. Eating more light protein, fruit, vegetables, and fiber, while cutting out fatty and sugary foods, may help reduce cellulite.

FOOD	TYPICAL SERVING SIZE	FIBER CONTENT (IN GRAMS)
Beans & Legumes		
Beans, kidney, red, canned	½ cup	8
Peas, split, boiled	½ cup	8
Lentils, boiled	½ cup	8
Beans, black, boiled	½ cup	7.5
Beans, pinto, boiled	½ cup	7.5
Lima beans, boiled	½ cup	6.5
Beans, kidney, red, boiled	½ cup	6.5
Beans, baked, canned, plain or vegetarian	½ cup	6.5
Beans, white, canned	½ cup	6.5
Vegetables (Other)		
Artichokes, boiled	1 cup	9
Peas, boiled	1 cup	9
Vegetables, mixed, boiled	1 cup	8
Lettuce, iceberg	1 head	7.5
Pumpkin, canned	1 cup	7
Brussels sprouts, frozen, boiled	1 cup	6
Parsnips, boiled	1 cup	6
Turnip greens, boiled	1 cup	5
Potato, baked with skin	1 medium	3.8
Corn, yellow, cooked	½ cup	2.3
Tomato, red, raw	1 large	2.2
Carrot, raw	1 medium	1.7

FOOD	TYPICAL SERVING SIZE	FIBER CONTENT (IN GRAMS)
Starches		
All-Bran Extra Fiber (Kellogg's)	1 cup	15
Fiber One (General Mills)	1 cup	14
Granola, homemade	1 cup	13
All-Bran (Kellogg's)	1 cup	9.7
Bulgur wheat, cooked	1 cup	8
Raisin Bran (Kellogg's)	1 cup	8
100% Bran (Post)	1 cup	8.3
Bran Chex (Kellogg's); Multi-Bran Chex (General Mills)	1 cup	8
Shredded Wheat; Wheat 'n Bran (Post)	1¼ cups	8
Oat bran, cooked	½ cup	6
Spaghetti, whole-wheat	½ cup	3
Oatmeal	½ cup	2
Bread, whole-wheat	1 slice	2
Bread, mixed-grain	1 slice	1.8
Rice, brown	½ cup	1.8
Bread, cracked-wheat	1 slice	1.6
Bread, rye	1 slice	1.6
Fruits		
Raspberries, frozen, unsweetened	1 cup	17
Prunes, stewed, unsweetened	1 cup	16
Raspberries, raw	1 cup	8
Pear	1 fruit	5.5

FOOD	TYPICAL SERVING SIZE	FIBER CONTENT (IN GRAMS)
Avocado, Florida	¼ fruit	4.5
Blueberries, raw	1 cup	7.6
Papaya, whole	1 fruit	5.5
Figs, dried	2 figs	4.6
Apple	1 medium	3.3
Banana	1 medium	3.1
Orange	1 medium	3.1
Strawberries, whole	1 cup	3
Peach	1 medium	2.2

Source: Nutrient Data Laboratory. USDA Nutrient Database for Standard Reference

FOR OVERALL FAT BURNING

The Zumba Diet program is not so much a diet per se, but an eating philosophy that helps you lose fat. It emphasizes fresh, whole foods that are minimally processed, lean, and organic whenever possible. The food is delicious, good for you, and you will lose weight steadily without feeling deprived. Because the diet is based on high-fiber foods like fruits, vegetables, and whole grains, you tend to feel satisfied on fewer calories. Keep these tips in mind, too:

✳ Always eat breakfast. It revs up your metabolism for the day.

✳ Do not skimp on protein. Your body has to work harder to digest protein than it does carbs, burning up more calories. Aim for three good servings a day. The omega-3 fats in fish help reduce the size of fat cells in the body; have at least two servings of fish a week.

✳ Opt for mostly resistant starches as your starch choices: beans, bananas (slightly green), yams, potatoes, barley, brown rice, and corn.

✳ Veg out. Eat unlimited vegetables (excluding potatoes, corn, peas, and other starchy vegetables) to keep your metabolism raised for minimal calories. Have at least three servings a day. Also include two to three servings of fruit a day.

✳ Do not skip meals. If your body gets used to not eating for long stretches, it will adapt by conserving energy and reducing the number of calories it burns. It is a bad idea regularly to "save yourself" for a big dinner by eating nothing during the day. Your metabolism will go into starvation mode and your body will burn up fewer of the calories you eat that evening.

✳ Snack smart. Eating often keeps your burn rate up. Time your snacks to eat before and after exercise. Try to combine the food groups, always including a protein and a starch or fruit.

Zumba Fitness has created three specific fourteen-day meal plans that show you how to put targeted dieting into action. You will find them in the next chapter.

HOW TO STRUCTURE YOUR MEALS

While on the Zumba Diet, you eat three main meals a day and two snacks *on the days you exercise*—a pre-exercise snack and a post-exercise snack.

It is essential that you have both a light protein and a starch at each main meal, with a vegetable and/or a fruit tossed in. You will also be able to enjoy a little healthy fat—up to two servings a day. The light protein and starch are two key elements in your meals. Protein slows the rate at which starches are digested. This combination of foods helps regulate your blood sugar level, to fuel your muscles, and to give you a steady release of energy throughout the day to support your activities, including Zumba. It also curbs cravings for sweets.

I am sure many of you are thinking: light proteins, starches, and vegetables—you call that tasty?

If you look over the food lists on the previous pages and note the variety, and if you study the meal plans in the next chapter, you will realize that this way of eating is not only appetizing, but satisfying. Then, after only a few days of eating like this, check your energy level and mood. I am sure you will feel better than you have in a long time. Of course, let me emphasize again and again: eating high-quality food like this will help you lose weight more efficiently and enhance your body shape.

Breakfast, Lunch, and Dinner

It is also important to learn what makes a balanced meal. Here is how the perfect plate should look: One-third protein, about the size of your palm—a chicken breast, for example; one-third starch, such as rice, pasta, or potatoes; and one-third high-volume vegetables. Reserve fruit for breakfast, snacks, or dessert. But have two to three fruits a day. For breakfast, you would not ordinarily eat vegetables, so the balance should change to one-third protein, such as two scrambled egg whites; one-third starch, such as oatmeal or a slice of whole-grain toast, and a fruit.

Pre-Exercise Snacks

On the days you exercise, it is important to fuel yourself before and after your workout. The goal of a pre-exercise snack is to energize you for exercise. The food eaten before a workout not only gets burned for fuel but helps to maintain a normal blood sugar. You will want to eat a small snack two to three hours before your workout. This snack should include a fresh fruit or starch (if not eaten at your main meal) and a small portion of protein. Remember, protein slows the absorption of carbohydrates to help maintain steady, evenly released blood sugar. Nuts, which are technically a fat, contain protein, so they make great snacks on this plan.

Post-Exercise Snacks

After exercising, your muscles need some repair and rebuilding time, so it is wise to nourish yourself following your workout. One of the most effective ways to do this is to eat immediately after a workout. During this period, your muscles are most receptive to replenishing their energy reserves, so a snack within fifteen to thirty minutes after your workout provides a real boost. Include a little protein in your snack to help your muscles repair faster.

Snack Suggestions

* Slice of whole-grain bread (if not eaten at a main meal) + a slice of low-fat cheese

* Piece of fresh fruit + hard-boiled egg

* 1 banana + 1 cup fat-free, no-sugar yogurt

* Smoothie: 1 cup frozen unsweetened berries blended with 1 cup skim or nondairy milk, or 1 cup of nonfat yogurt

* Cottage cheese + fresh fruit

* Slice of cheese + raw veggies

* Piece of fresh fruit + 1 hard-boiled egg

* Cup of low-sodium or fresh vegetable juice + 8 walnuts

* Piece of fresh fruit + 12 almonds

* Medium baked potato + 2 ounces of light protein

* Energy bar or drink containing protein and carbohydrate (150 calories or less per serving)

A QUICK & EASY OVERVIEW OF THE ZUMBA DIET

Breakfast	1 light protein + 1 starch + 1 fruit
Lunch	1 light protein + 1 starch + high-volume vegetables
Dinner	1 light protein + 1 starch + high-volume vegetables
Pre-Exercise Snack	1 small portion of light protein + 1 starch or 1 fruit or high-volume vegetable (on workout days)
Post-Exercise Snack	1 small portion of light protein + 1 starch or 1 fruit or high-volume vegetable (on workout days)
Healthy Fats	Up to 2 servings a day

DETERMINING HOW MUCH FOOD TO EAT

Though the Zumba Diet is full of good-for-you foods, it does not give you license to eat as much as you want. You need to watch your portion sizes.

But in true Zumba fashion, there will be nothing to weigh and nothing to measure, unless you want to or you desire to be very precise. All of the things you need to estimate your portions are with you all the time. A regular teaspoon, a tablespoon, a glass, a bowl, or a cup are common items on every table. Where it says a cup, it means a standard teacup, the kind sitting in your cupboard right now. Where a meal says a slice, this refers to a standard slice such as you find in a loaf of bread, or sliced cheese. And if you divide your plate as I described above, you will automatically serve up the right amount of food. The number of calories takes care of itself.

But in most cases, your measuring device will be your hand. The standard guideline we use for men and women is: your light protein (such as a piece of lean meat) should be able to fit in the palm of your hand, your starch portion should be able to fit in your cupped hand, and your fat portion should be the size of your thumb. High-volume vegetables can be eaten in unlimited quantities. As for fruits, one piece of fruit is a serving. A serving of berries or cut-up fresh fruit would be about the size of your fist.

If you are a woman standing five feet tall, do not feel cheated when you compare the palm of your hand with that of your boyfriend or husband, who might be taller or heavier than you are. Yes, he has a bigger palm, and he gets to eat more, but that's by design.

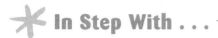

✳ In Step With . . .

Marcella Allen, Los Angeles, California

Marcella has a heart for the less fortunate. Once a week, she teaches Zumba on a volunteer basis at an inner-city church that provides various services to the surrounding disadvantaged neighborhood. Two Saturdays a month, she teaches the class to the elementary school children and teen girls. And she teaches Zumba at a shelter for women protected from domestic abuse.

"These experiences are the most rewarding," says Marcella, a former ballroom dancer. "The looks on their faces when the music comes up is absolutely priceless. While they dance, they leave their world behind to have fun."

Marcella became trained and licensed as a Zumba Fitness instructor in 2008. In addition to teaching at a gym, she saw opportunities to bring Zumba Fitness to those in need of uplifting. Zumba is now her passion, and she's spreading it around.

CONDIMENTS AND EXTRAS: SPICE UP YOUR FOOD

I like to be realistic: A salad without dressing or a baked potato with no sour cream leaves a lot to be desired. But while condiments add zip to food, they often contain tons of calories, fat, and sugar. Here are some ways to spice up your food without adding unhealthy extras.

* Use spices and herbs, particularly sodium-free or reduced-sodium products. By adding spices and herbs, you can boost significant levels of health-promoting antioxidants in just about any dish on the table. Some of the best spices to use include cinnamon, ginger, oregano, basil, red peppers (including cayenne, crushed red pepper, and paprika), rosemary, yellow curry, and thyme.

✳ Go easy on ketchup. It has around eighty calories per tablespoon. It is also high in sodium, and many products are loaded with sugar. As an alternative to regular ketchup, try no-sugar or low-carb versions.

✳ Great alternatives to ketchup are steak sauce, unsweetened relish, hot sauces, and salsa. However, these alternatives do contain a significant amount of sodium, so don't overdo them.

✳ Use mustard. It has minimal calories and fat, no sugar, and is low in sodium. One tablespoon has only ten calories and zero grams of fat, making it a good alternative to full-fat mayonnaise on sandwiches. Dijon mustard, in particular, pairs well with baked chicken breasts. There are many types of mustard available. Avoid honey mustards, however, which are high in sugar.

✳ If you want to add some flavor to your salad with even less fat, salad spritzers may be the perfect solution. These products are sold in seven-ounce bottles and supply lots of flavor to salads with very little fat or calories.

✳ Any oil-free salad dressing is allowed in reasonable amounts.

✳ All vinegars are allowed.

✳ For cutting down on fat, try fat-free mayonnaise. Most people cannot even tell the difference between this mayonnaise and the real thing.

✳ Try fat-free foods such as fat-free sour cream, fat-free cream cheese, and nonfat whipped topping, as well as sugar-free condiments in moderate amounts.

✳ Low-carb and sugar-free condiments are allowed, too: light pancake syrup, reduced-sugar jam, and artificial sweeteners, all in moderation.

✳ Nonstick vegetable spray and artificial sweeteners are permitted, too, within moderation.

✳ Certain desserts are included on the Zumba Diet—up to three servings a week of the dessert recipes created for the diet. (See pages 268–269.)

PERMISSIBLE BEVERAGES

The number-one beverage to drink is water (tap, bottled, carbonated, and sodium-free car-bonated water). Water is paramount to dieting: it can actually jack up your body's fat-burning mechanism.

Water carries both the nutrients our body needs to function and the waste produced by cellular metabolism. Without it, the body becomes chronically dehydrated and vulnerable to illness. Drink as much water as you can throughout the day. It will help to rid your system of toxins, combat bloating, and improve the look of your skin and hair. You need at least six to eight cups a day—and eight to ten cups on the days when you participate in Zumba.

Also, start each day with a cup of warm water with a squeeze of fresh lemon juice, and drink before breakfast. It will go straight through to the bowels, flushing out mucus and toxins fast, as well as helping the body to rehydrate.

Other permissible beverages on the Zumba Diet include:

✳ Coffee, tea, green tea, and herbal tea. I highly recommend green tea, in particular. Some of the antioxidants it contains may slightly speed up fat-burning, according to recent studies. It also has appetite-suppressive effects. Moreover, green tea does not seem to raise heart rates, which could make it a more effective stimulant for overweight people with high blood pressure or heart disease.

✳ Low-sodium or fresh vegetable juices (tomato juice, vegetable juice, carrot juice)—up to one cup or eight ounces a day. Vegetable juices are an excellent way to increase your vegetable intake. Some products contain sodium, so opt for reduced-sodium versions.

A caution: It is best to avoid alcoholic beverages while you are focused on losing weight. They are full of calories, easily metabolized into fat, and will lower your inhibitions, making it more difficult to stay the course.

Now, if you are ready to drop pounds, alter your shape, and feel energized, let's move on to the next chapter and see how to start planning meals for great results.

Chapter 11
MEAL MAGIC

The Zumba Diet is really three diets in one: the Zumba Basic Diet, the Zumba Flat Abs Diet, and the Zumba Thin Thighs Diet. Each plan includes fourteen days of menus as a guideline for how to eat and includes a variety of delicious recipes from Chapter 12. You can follow the sample meal plans here or you can map out your own meals using the food lists, guidelines, and the Zumba Meal Planner on page 234.

Using sample meals can make things easier for you, especially when you begin the plan. Let them just be a helpful guide, but do not allow them to restrict you. If you do not like some of the food items on the sample menus, do not force yourself to eat them. If you hate tuna fish, for example, then come up with a different light protein you do like. Forcing yourself to eat foods you dislike is a shortcut to failure.

No matter which plan you decide to follow, this chapter shows you exactly what to eat and how to eat. There are really no hard and fast rules here, except one: Enjoy your meals!

14-DAY ZUMBA BASIC DIET

This plan shows you how to put together meals for maximum nutrition and weight loss and provides a general guide for how to eat each day. Remember, you can follow it exactly as written, or adapt it to your own food preferences. Also, there are recipes in Chapter 12 that correspond to some of the suggestions in this diet. This plan provides a strategy that encourages overall weight loss and harnesses the power of protein and resistant starch to help you rid yourself of unwanted pounds.

DAY 1

Breakfast

½ cup *Low-Fat, Low-Sugar Granola* (page 246), sprinkled with 8 walnuts, crushed

1 cup nondairy milk

1 banana, sliced

Green tea or coffee

Lunch

Chicken breast, grilled or baked

½ cup commercial bean salad, drained and served over lettuce leaves

1 piece of fresh fruit

Dinner

Lamb chops, grilled

1 medium sweet potato, baked

Brussels sprouts, steamed or boiled

Pre- and Post-Exercise Snacks

1 energy bar or nutrition drink

1 cup fat-free, no-sugar, fruit-flavored yogurt + 1 piece fresh fruit

DAY 2

Breakfast

1 egg, scrambled

1 slice whole-wheat toast

½ grapefruit or other fruit in season

Green tea or coffee

Lunch

Broiled cheese sandwich: 2 slices cheddar cheese and one slice of tomato on one slice of cracked-wheat bread, broiled

1 bowl *Garden Vegetable Soup* (page 249)

Dinner

Saucy Salmon (page 261)

½ cup *Greek Barley Salad* (page 254)

Broccoli, boiled or steamed

Pre- and Post-Exercise Snacks

1 energy bar or nutrition drink

Smoothie: 1 cup frozen unsweetened berries blended with 1 cup of skim milk or nondairy milk

DAY 3

Breakfast

Turkey bacon, two slices, cooked

½ cup oat bran or other hot whole-grain cereal

1 cup fresh berries

Lunch

Bowl of *Ajiaco* (page 250)

1 cup fat-free, no-sugar, fruit-flavored yogurt

Dinner

Sirloin steak, broiled or grilled

Twice-Baked Garlic Cheese Potatoes (page 257)

Tossed salad: 2 cups leaf lettuce, 1 green pepper (chopped), ½ cup raw shredded carrot, ¼ cup chopped onion, 2 tablespoons salad dressing (any type)

Pre- and Post-Exercise Snacks

1 energy bar or nutrition drink

¼ cup cottage cheese + 1 piece of fresh fruit

DAY 4

Breakfast

1 cup fat-free, no-sugar, fruit-flavored yogurt mixed with ½ cup *Low-Fat, Low-Sugar Granola* (page 246)

1 pear, sliced

Lunch

Quick-Fix Fajitas (page 260)

1 orange

Dinner

Turkey breast, baked or grilled

Sweet Potato Fruit Purée (page 258)

Vegetable medley (broccoli, carrots, cauliflower), boiled or steamed

Pre- and Post-Exercise Snacks

1 apple + 12 almonds (raw or roasted without oil)

1 cup fat-free, no-sugar, fruit-flavored yogurt + 1 piece fresh fruit

---

DAY 5

Breakfast

Cinnamon Raisin French Toast (page 246), with 1 tablespoon light pancake syrup

1 banana, sliced

Lunch

Tofu Lasagna (page 264)

1 plum or other fresh fruit in season

Dinner

Quick Rosemary Pork Chops, 2 (page 264)

½ cup low-fat creamed corn

Asparagus, boiled or steamed—or other green vegetable

Pre- and Post-Exercise Snacks

Baby carrots + 1 slice low-fat cheese

1 cup fat-free, no-sugar, fruit-flavored yogurt + 1 piece fresh fruit

DAY 6

Breakfast

½ cup oatmeal, cooked

1 cup nondairy milk

1 fresh peach, sliced

Lunch

Southwestern Lettuce Wraps (page 260)

1 orange

Dinner

Chicken thighs, baked or grilled, topped with 2 tablespoons salsa

½ cup pinto beans

Tossed salad: 2 cups leaf lettuce, 1 green pepper (chopped), ½ cup raw shredded carrot, ¼ cup chopped onion, 2 tablespoons salad dressing (any type)

1 serving *Luscious Key Lime Pie* (page 268)

Pre- and Post-Exercise Snacks

1 energy bar or nutrition drink

1 cup fat-free, no-sugar, fruit-flavored yogurt + 1 banana, sliced

DAY 7

Breakfast

Turkey sausage patties, 2

½ cup Cream of Wheat, or other cooked whole-grain cereal

½ grapefruit

Lunch

1 bowl of lentil soup

2 ounces cheese

Tossed salad: 2 cups leaf lettuce, 1 green pepper (chopped), ½ cup raw shredded carrot, ¼ cup chopped onion, 2 tablespoons salad dressing (any type)

Dinner

Salmon, grilled or baked

½ cup brown rice, cooked

Green Bean Casserole (page 256)

1 serving *Cherry Cheesecake* (page 269)

Pre- and Post-Exercise Snacks

1 energy bar or nutrition drink

1 cup skim or nondairy milk + 1 piece fresh fruit

DAY 8

Breakfast

½ cup oat bran, cooked

1 egg, poached, hard-boiled, or scrambled

1 banana, sliced

Green tea or coffee

Lunch

Marinated Garbanzo Bean Salad (page 255)

Dinner

Meat and Rice Loaf (page 267)

Caesar salad: 1 cup chopped romaine lettuce, 6 tablespoons shredded raw carrot, ½ cup chopped cucumber, and 2 tablespoons fat-free Caesar salad dressing

Pre- and Post-Exercise Snacks

1 energy bar or nutrition drink

1 cup fat-free, no-sugar, fruit-flavored yogurt + 1 piece fresh fruit

DAY 9

Breakfast

½ cup oatmeal, cooked

1 cup fat-free, no-sugar, fruit-flavored yogurt

1 cup fresh cherries, or other fruit in season

Green tea or coffee

Lunch

Water-packed tuna with one sliced tomato, ½ cup cannelini beans, served on a generous bed of lettuce, drizzled with 2 tablespoons *Zesty Olive Oil Vinaigrette* (page 252)

Dinner

1 baked Cornish game hen, skin removed

½ cup bulgur wheat, cooked, or ½ cup brown rice

Carrots, boiled or steamed

1 cup melon balls, or other fresh fruit

Pre- and Post-Exercise Snacks

1 energy bar or drink

¼ cup low-fat cottage cheese + raw cut-up veggies

DAY 10

Breakfast

Western Omelet (page 247)

½ cup corn grits, cooked

1 cup fresh berries

Green tea or coffee

Lunch

Hummus: ½ cup garbanzo beans (puréed and mixed with 1 tablespoon olive oil), 1 tomato (sliced). Served on cucumber slices

½ cup low-fat cottage cheese

Dinner

Sesame Fish (page 263)

½ cup *Coconut Rice* (page 259)

Caesar salad: 2 cups shredded romaine lettuce, 1 chopped tomato, 2 tablespoons chopped onion, 1 grated carrot, and 2 tablespoons Caesar salad dressing

Pre- and Post-Exercise Snacks

1 energy bar or nutrition drink

1 cup fat-free, no-sugar, fruit-flavored yogurt + 1 banana, sliced

DAY 11

Breakfast

½ cup *Low-Fat, Low-Sugar Granola* (page 246)

1 cup nondairy milk

1 banana, sliced

Lunch

Chicken breast, grilled

1 bowl *White Bean Soup* (page 248)

1 cup fat-free, no-sugar, fruit-flavored yogurt

Dinner

Extra-lean hamburger patty, broiled or grilled

1 ear of corn, boiled

Broccoli, steamed

Pre- and Post-Exercise Snacks

1 cup (8 ounces) vegetable or tomato juice + 12 almonds or 8 walnuts

1 cup fat-free, no-sugar, fruit-flavored yogurt + 1 piece fresh fruit

DAY 12

Breakfast

Western Omelet (page 247)

1 slice whole-wheat toast

½ grapefruit or other fresh fruit in season

Lunch

½ cup low-fat cottage cheese served on a baked potato with bacon bits

1 bowl *Garden Vegetable Soup* (page 249)

Cali Fruit Slaw (page 255)

Dinner

2 lamb chops, broiled or grilled

1 medium sweet potato, baked

Green beans, boiled or steamed

1 serving *Cherry Cheesecake* (page 269)

Pre- and Post-Exercise Snacks

1 cup (8 ounces) vegetable or tomato juice + 12 almonds or 8 walnuts

1 cup fat-free, no-sugar, fruit-flavored yogurt + 1 piece fresh fruit

DAY 13

Breakfast

1 cup high-fiber cereal

1 cup nondairy milk or skim milk

Peach, sliced

Lunch

Gourmet Spinach Salad (page 253)

Dinner

Miami Crab Cakes (page 262)

½ cup brown rice, cooked

Marinated Vegetable Medley (page 254)

1 serving *Luscious Key Lime Pie* (page 268)

Pre- and Post-Exercise Snacks

1 nutrition drink or bar

Strawberry Shake (page 272)

DAY 14

Breakfast

Peachy Shake (page 270)

Lunch

Tuna Nicoise Salad (page 252)

Dinner

Barbecued Steak (page 267)

Fried Zucchini (page 256)

½ cup corn

14-DAY ZUMBA FLAT ABS DIET

There are certain foods that help to reduce belly fat, and these bodyshaping foods are incorporated into this version of the Zumba Diet. On this plan, you will pack your diet with soy, fish, yogurt and other calcium-rich foods, whole grains, and monounsaturated fats. You should also cut out trans fats completely; they may increase belly size.

DAY 1

Breakfast

1 cup fat-free, no-sugar, fruit-flavored yogurt

1 slice whole-wheat bread with a tablespoon of peanut butter

½ grapefruit

Green tea or coffee

Lunch

1 whole-wheat pita stuffed with hummus (about 4–5 tablespoons), 3 slices tomato, 1 slice red onion, and chopped salad greens

½ cup calcium-fortified low-fat cottage cheese

1 apple

Dinner

Sesame Fish (page 263)

½ cup brown rice, cooked

Carrots, boiled or steamed

Pre- and Post-Exercise Snacks

1 cup (8 ounces) vegetable or tomato juice + 1 slice cheese

1 cup fat-free, no-sugar, fruit-flavored yogurt + 1 piece fresh fruit

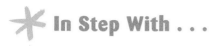 **In Step With . . .**

Karley Abramson, Orchard Lake, Michigan

Like many women, Karley, a college student, struggled with liking herself. "It's not easy being a young woman in today's world, with the plethora of absurd and ultimately dangerous standards of beauty staring us down at every corner," she states. "For years, I tried desperately to retain the last few threads of self-worth that the size-0 supermodels on the covers of magazines had not taken from me, but holding on has been like trying to hold on to water in cupped hands. It's almost impossible to maintain positive self-esteem."

Not only was Karley's self-esteem breaking apart, so was her family life. By her senior year in college, there were problems between her mother and father. Karley's self-worth sank to an all-time low.

Her emotional lifeline came in the form of Zumba. As a college senior, Karley began to teach Zumba to college students at the University of Michigan. At first the classes were small, but by the second semester her classes were packed, and students were standing in line to get into her class. "I had developed a loyal following of die-hard Zumba groupies." She smiles.

There was no time for Karley to be down in the dumps over her family's plight. "When the reality of my family crisis hit, Zumba was the cushion I fell back on," she says. "If I sank into a depression, Zumba was the only thing that gave me the strength and energy to leave my room. Who was I to hide out under the covers of my bed when there were fifty girls ready to continue the party? Many of these girls depended on me to get them through their week. In retrospect, I now realize how desperately I needed them to get me through mine. Zumba became my personal medication, and continues to be my savior today."

Every student smiled and laughed through every sweaty class. They kept coming back for more. "Their support boosted my self-esteem in a way that nothing else ever had," Karley recalls. "Not only was I feeling better from exercising regularly (it's true about those endorphins), but I also could see how my class buoyed the self-esteem of many other young college women as well.

"Our Zumba class is a place where we can all gather and let loose: no competitiveness, no gossiping, and no judgment crossing the threshold. We are just young girls getting our groove on in a safe haven, momentarily free from the pressures and stresses of the outside world.

"Had I not discovered Zumba during those few months prior to my family crisis, I honestly do not know what state I would be in today."

DAY 2

Breakfast

1 cup fat-free, no-sugar, fruit-flavored yogurt

1 slice whole-wheat bread, toasted, with
2 teaspoons reduced-sugar jam

1 orange, medium

Green tea or coffee

Lunch

Open-face egg salad sandwich: Mix one
hard-boiled egg with 1 tablespoon olive
oil and 1 teaspoon of yellow prepared
mustard. Place on one slice of whole-wheat
bread and top with ½ cup alfalfa sprouts

1 bowl *Spicy Tomato Soup* (page 249)

Dinner

Scallop Kabobs (page 263)

Sweet Potato Fruit Purée (page 258)

1 tomato, sliced—drizzle with 1 tablespoon
red wine vinegar and 1 tablespoon olive oil

Pre- and Post-Exercise Snacks

1 energy bar or nutrition drink

1 cup fat-free, no-sugar, fruit-flavored
yogurt + 1 piece fresh fruit

DAY 3

Breakfast

1 cup high-fiber cereal

1 cup nondairy milk

1 cup fresh blueberries (or other fruit in
season)

Green tea or coffee

Lunch

Chicken thighs, baked or grilled—sprinkle
with walnut pieces (8 walnuts chopped)

1 bowl *Garden Vegetable Soup* (page 249),
with ½ cup cooked barley

1 orange

Dinner

Meat and Rice Loaf (page 267)

Caesar salad: 1 cup chopped romaine
lettuce, 6 tablespoons shredded raw
carrot, ½ cup chopped cucumber,
and 2 tablespoons fat-free Caesar
salad dressing

Pre- and Post-Exercise Snacks

1 energy bar or nutrition drink

1 apple + 1 cup fat-free, no-sugar,
fruit-flavored yogurt

DAY 4

Breakfast

½ cup oat bran, cooked

1 cup nondairy milk

1 cup fresh strawberries

Green tea or coffee

Lunch

Crab salad: lump crabmeat served over
¼ avocado, 1 chopped tomato, onion
slices, and lettuce. Drizzle with
2 tablespoons balsamic vinegar and
1 tablespoon olive or canola oil

½ cup brown rice, cooked

1 orange

Dinner

Tofu Lasagna (page 264)

Tossed salad: 2 cups leaf lettuce,
1 green pepper (chopped), ½ cup raw
shredded carrot, ¼ cup chopped onion,
2 tablespoons fat-free salad dressing

Pre- and Post-Exercise Snacks

1 energy bar or nutrition drink

1 apple + 1 cup fat-free, no-sugar, fruit-
flavored yogurt

DAY 5

Breakfast

1 cup high-fiber cereal

1 cup nondairy milk

½ grapefruit

Green tea or coffee

Lunch

Gourmet Spinach Salad (page 253)

1 cup fat-free, no-sugar, fruit-flavored
yogurt

1 piece fresh fruit in season

Dinner

Chicken breast (skin removed), baked
or grilled

½ cup bulgur wheat

Carrots, steamed or boiled

Pre- and Post-Exercise Snacks

1 energy bar or nutrition drink

1 apple + 1 cup fat-free, no-sugar,
fruit-flavored yogurt

DAY 6

Breakfast

Berry Soy Shake (page 270)

½ cup oatmeal, cooked

Green tea or coffee

Lunch

1 bowl *Spicy Tomato Soup* (page 249)

2 ounces soy cheese

1 slice mixed-grain bread

Dinner

Grilled or steamed shrimp, with 3 tablespoons cocktail sauce

½ cup corn, cooked

Tossed salad: 2 cups leaf lettuce, 1 green pepper (chopped), ½ cup raw shredded carrot, ¼ cup chopped onion, 1 tablespoon olive oil salad dressing

1 serving *Cherry Cheesecake* (page 269)

Pre- and Post-Exercise Snacks

1 energy bar or nutrition drink

1 apple + 1 cup fat-free, no-sugar, fruit-flavored yogurt

DAY 7

Breakfast

1 egg, scrambled

½ cup corn grits, cooked

½ grapefruit

Green tea or coffee

Lunch

Chicken breast (skin removed), baked or broiled

½ cup couscous, cooked

Marinated Vegetable Medley (page 254)

1 cup fat-free, no-sugar, fruit-flavored yogurt

Dinner

Tangy Catfish Creole (page 263)

½ cup brown rice, cooked

Green beans, boiled or steamed

¼ avocado, sliced, drizzled with 1 tablespoon red wine vinegar and 1½ teaspoons olive oil

1 serving *Luscious Key Lime Pie* (page 268)

Pre- and Post-Exercise Snacks

1 energy bar or nutrition drink

1 cup (8 ounces) vegetable or tomato juice + 12 almonds

DAY 8

Breakfast

½ cup *Low-Fat, Low-Sugar Granola* (page 246)

1 cup nondairy milk

1 cup fresh strawberries (or other berries)

Green tea or coffee

Lunch

Water-packed tuna with one sliced tomato served on a generous bed of lettuce

1 slice cracked-wheat bread

2 tablespoons *Zesty Olive Oil Vinaigrette* (page 252)

Dinner

Turkey breast, baked

1 medium yam, baked

Asparagus spears, boiled or steamed

Pre- and Post-Exercise Snacks

1 energy bar or nutrition drink

1 piece fresh fruit + 1 cup fat-free, no-sugar, fruit-flavored yogurt

DAY 9

Breakfast

1 cup fat-free, no-sugar, fruit-flavored yogurt

1 slice mixed-grain bread

¼ melon or other fresh fruit in season

Green tea or coffee

Lunch

No-Carb Pizza (page 266)

Dinner

Easiest Salmon Ever (page 262)

½ cup *Dilled Rice* (page 259)

Broccoli (or other high-volume vegetable), boiled or steamed

Pre- and Post-Exercise Snacks

1 energy bar or nutrition drink

1 apple + 12 almonds or 8 walnuts

DAY 10

Breakfast

½ cup oat bran, cooked

1 cup nondairy milk

1 fresh peach, sliced

Green tea or coffee

Lunch

Gourmet Spinach Salad (page 253)

1 slice cracked-wheat bread

Dinner

Quick Rosemary Pork Chops (page 264)

½ cup green peas

Cauliflower, boiled or steamed

Pre- and Post-Exercise Snacks

1 energy bar or nutrition drink

1 apple with 2 tablespoons peanut butter

DAY 11

Breakfast

1 cup high-fiber cereal

1 cup nondairy milk

½ grapefruit

Green tea or coffee

Lunch

Turkey breast, baked or grilled

1 medium baked potato, topped with fat-free sour cream

Brussels sprouts, boiled or steamed

Dinner

Cod or other fish, baked or grilled

½ cup brown rice

Caesar salad: 2 cups shredded romaine lettuce, 1 chopped tomato, 2 tablespoons chopped onion, 1 grated carrot, and 2 tablespoons Caesar salad dressing

Pre- and Post-Exercise Snacks

1 energy bar or nutrition drink

1 banana + 1 cup fat-free, no-sugar, fruit flavored yogurt

DAY 12

Breakfast

½ cup *Low-Fat, Low-Sugar Granola* (page 246)

1 cup nondairy milk

1 cup fresh strawberries (or other seasonal fruit)

Green tea or coffee

Lunch

Chicken, baked or grilled

½ cup brown rice

Tossed salad: 2 cups leaf lettuce, 1 green pepper (chopped), ½ cup raw shredded carrot, ¼ cup chopped onion, 1 tablespoon olive oil salad dressing

Dinner

Carne Asada *with Colombian Green Sauce* (page 265)

½ cup whole-wheat pasta tossed with 1 tablespoon pine nuts and 2 tablespoons fat-free Parmesan cheese

Zucchini, boiled or steamed

Pre- and Post-Exercise Snacks

1 energy bar or nutrition drink

1 apple + 1 cup fat-free, no-sugar, fruit-flavored yogurt

DAY 13

Breakfast

Western Omelet (page 247)

1 slice whole-wheat bread, toasted

1 banana

Green tea or coffee

Lunch

Low-fat chef salad: 1 ounce fat-free cheddar cheese, 2 slices low-fat turkey ham, 1 chopped tomato, ½ cup raw broccoli, 2 cups lettuce, ¼ avocado, and 2 tablespoons fat-free French dressing

½ cup brown rice

Dinner

2 pork chops, baked or grilled

1 medium sweet potato, baked, or 1 cup mashed winter squash

Cauliflower, boiled or steamed

Colombian Mango Dessert (page 269)

Pre- and Post-Exercise Snacks

1 energy bar or nutrition drink

¼ cup low-fat cottage cheese + 1 cup chopped fresh pineapple

DAY 14

Breakfast

½ cup oatmeal, cooked

Rise and Shine Smoothie (page 271)

1 cup fresh cherries, or other fruit
in season

Green tea or coffee

Lunch

Fruit salad: ½ cup low-fat cottage cheese
on 2 pear halves and 1 cup chopped
lettuce leaves, 8 walnuts, chopped

1 slice multigrain bread

Dinner

1 Cornish game hen, skin removed, baked

Carrots, boiled or steamed

½ cup bulgur wheat, cooked, or ½ cup
brown rice, cooked

Cherry Cheesecake (page 269)

Pre- and Post-Exercise Snacks

1 energy bar or nutrition drink

Strawberry Shake (page 272)

14-DAY ZUMBA THIN THIGHS DIET

Fiber has earned a reputation as a fat fighter. Now research tells us that it helps trim fat from the thighs, which is why this version of the Zumba Diet is high in healthy fiber. This diet also incorporates other bodyshaping foods that, along with exercise, will help remodel your body.

DAY 1

Breakfast

- 1 cup high-fiber cereal
- 1 cup skim milk
- 1 fresh pear, sliced
- Green tea or coffee

Lunch

- *Tuna Nicoise Salad* (page 252)

Dinner

- Chicken breast, baked or grilled (skin removed, top with 2 tablespoons salsa)
- Brussel sprouts, boiled or steamed
- ½ cup pinto beans, cooked

Pre- and Post-Exercise Snacks

- 1 energy bar or nutrition drink
- ¼ cup cottage cheese + raw, cut-up veggies

DAY 2

Breakfast

- *Tropical Refresher* (page 271)
- 1 slice high-fiber wheat bread, toasted, with 2 tablespoons reduced-sugar jam
- Green tea or coffee

Lunch

- Black bean chili: ½ cup cooked black beans, ½ cup ground turkey, 1 cup stewed chopped tomatoes, 2 tablespoons chopped fresh onions
- 1 cup fat-free, no-sugar, fruit-flavored yogurt

Dinner

- Broiled or grilled round steak
- 1 medium baked potato with skin, topped with fat-free sour cream
- Tossed salad with assorted salad vegetables, 2 tablespoons French dressing

Pre- and Post-Exercise Snacks

- *Strawberry Shake* (page 272)
- 1 apple + 12 almonds or 8 walnuts

DAY 3

Breakfast

½ cup oat bran, cooked

1 egg, poached, hard-boiled, or scrambled

1 fresh peach

Green tea or coffee

Lunch

Gourmet Spinach Salad (page 253)

Dinner

Salmon Chowder (page 251)

½ cup brown rice, cooked

Artichoke Heart Salad (page 253)

Pre- and Post-Exercise Snacks

1 cup fat-free, no-sugar, fruit-flavored yogurt + 1 banana, sliced

1 cup low-sodium or fresh vegetable juice + 1 slice cheese

DAY 4

Breakfast

1 egg, scrambled

1 slice high-fiber bread, toasted

1 pear

Green tea or coffee

Lunch

Quick-Fix Fajitas (page 260)

2 tablespoons salsa

Dinner

Sesame Fish (page 263)

½ cup corn, cooked

Carrots, steamed or boiled

1 serving *Luscious Key Lime Pie* (page 268)

Pre- and Post-Exercise Snacks

1 energy bar or nutrition drink

1 apple + 12 almonds or 8 walnuts

DAY 5

Breakfast

   1 cup high-fiber cereal

   1 cup fresh berries

   1 cup skim milk

   Coffee or green tea

Lunch

   Marinated Garbanzo Bean Salad (page 255)

Dinner

   Ann's Easy Chicken (page 261)

   Asparagus spears, boiled or steamed

   ½ cup *Dilled Rice* (page 259)

Pre- and Post-Exercise Snacks

   1 energy bar or nutrition drink

   1 cup fat-free, no-sugar, fruit-flavored yogurt + 1 pear

DAY 6

Breakfast

   1 cup high-fiber cereal

   1 cup nondairy milk

   1 fresh orange

   Green tea or coffee

Lunch

   Leftover chicken

   1 bowl *White Bean Soup* (page 248)

   1 cup fat-free, no-sugar, fruit-flavored yogurt

Dinner

   Tuna steak, grilled

   1 medium potato, baked in skin, topped with fat-free sour cream

   Tossed salad: 2 cups leaf lettuce, 1 green pepper (chopped), ½ cup raw shredded carrot, ¼ cup chopped onion, 2 tablespoons French dressing

   Colombian Mango Dessert (page 269)

Pre- and Post-Exercise Snacks

   1 energy bar or nutrition drink

   1 cup fat-free, no-sugar, fruit flavored yogurt + 1 pear

DAY 7

Breakfast

1 cup high-fiber cereal

1 cup nondairy milk

½ grapefruit

Green tea or coffee

Lunch

Steamed shrimp

2 tablespoons cocktail sauce

½ cup corn, cooked

Cali Fruit Slaw (page 255)

Dinner

Quick Rosemary Pork Chops (page 264)

1 medium sweet potato, baked

Cauliflower, boiled or steamed

Pre- and Post-Exercise Snacks:

Chocolate Frappe (page 272)

1 apple or pear + 12 almonds or 8 walnuts

DAY 8

Breakfast

1 egg, scrambled

1 slice high-fiber wheat bread, toasted

½ cup stewed prunes, unsweetened,
or 1 fresh pear

Green tea or coffee

Lunch

Hummus: ½ cup garbanzo beans (puréed
and mixed with 1 tablespoon olive oil),
1 tomato, sliced, served on cucumber
slices

½ cup low-fat cottage cheese with
1 tomato, sliced

Dinner

Barbecued Steak (page 267)

1 medium potato, baked in skin, topped
with fat-free sour cream

Tossed salad: 2 cups leaf lettuce,
1 green pepper (chopped), ½ cup raw
shredded carrot, ¼ cup chopped onion,
2 tablespoons fat-free French dressing

Pre- and Post-Exercise Snacks

1 cup low-sodium or fresh vegetable juice
+ 1 slice cheese

1 cup fresh berries + 1 cup fat-free,
no-sugar, fruit-flavored yogurt

DAY 9

Breakfast

Peachy Shake (page 270)

Green tea or coffee

Lunch

Chicken Caesar salad: 2 cups shredded romaine lettuce, cubed grilled chicken breast, 2 tablespoons chopped onions, ½ chopped green pepper, 2 tablespoons Caesar salad dressing

1 slice high-fiber wheat bread

Dinner

Turkey breast, baked or grilled

1 cup winter squash, cooked and mashed

Green beans, boiled or steamed

1 serving *Cherry Cheesecake* (page 269)

Pre- and Post-Exercise Snacks

¼ cup cottage cheese + raw cut-up veggies

1 pear + 1 cup nondairy milk or skim milk

DAY 10

Breakfast

1 cup fat-free, no-sugar, fruit-flavored yogurt

1 slice high-fiber wheat bread, toasted

1 banana, sliced

Green tea or coffee

Lunch

Shrimp salad: Cooked shrimp (diced), 3 tablespoons chopped onion, 2 cups chopped lettuce, 1 tomato (large), and 1 tablespoon low-fat mayonnaise

½ cup corn, cooked

1 pear

Dinner

Easiest Salmon Ever (page 262)

1 medium sweet potato

Summer squash, boiled or steamed

Pre- and Post-Exercise Snacks

1 energy bar or nutrition drink

1 apple + 12 almonds or 8 walnuts

DAY 11

Breakfast

1 cup high-fiber cereal

1 cup nondairy milk

1 fresh orange

Green tea or coffee

Lunch

Miami Crab Cakes (page 262)

½ cup pinto beans, cooked

1 cup fresh berries

Dinner

Ann's Easy Chicken (page 261)

½ cup brown rice

Brussels sprouts, boiled or steamed

Pre- and Post-Exercise Snacks

1 energy bar or nutrition drink

1 banana + 1 cup nondairy milk or skim milk

DAY 12

Breakfast

½ cup oat-bran cereal, cooked

1 cup skim milk

1 cup diced mango, or 1 piece other seasonal fruit

Green tea or coffee

Lunch

Extra-lean hamburger patty

½ cup commercial three-bean salad, drained

Fried Zucchini (page 256)

Dinner

2 pork chops, baked or grilled

Acorn squash, baked (½ squash)

Green beans, steamed or boiled

Tossed salad: 2 cups leaf lettuce, 1 green pepper (chopped), ½ cup raw shredded carrot, ¼ cup chopped onion, 2 tablespoons French dressing

Pre- and Post-Exercise Snacks

1 energy bar or nutrition drink

¼ cup low-fat cottage cheese + raw cut-up veggies

DAY 13

Breakfast

Berry Soy Shake (page 270)

1 slice whole-wheat bread

Green tea or coffee

Lunch

Southwestern Lettuce Wraps (page 260)

1 pear or apple

Dinner

Sirloin steak, broiled or grilled

1 medium baked potato

Tossed salad: 2 cups leaf lettuce, 1 green pepper (chopped), ½ cup raw shredded carrot, ¼ cup chopped onion, 2 tablespoons salad dressing (any type)

Pre- and Post-Exercise Snacks

1 banana + 1 cup fat-free, no-sugar, fruit-flavored yogurt

1 slice cheese + raw cut-up veggies

DAY 14

Breakfast

Turkey sausage, 2 patties

½ cup cooked oat bran

½ grapefruit

Green tea or coffee

Lunch

½ cup cottage cheese served on tomato cut into wedges

1 bowl *Garden Vegetable Soup* (page 249)

1 slice high-fiber wheat bread

Dinner

Red snapper or other fish, grilled or baked

Caesar salad: 1 cup chopped romaine lettuce, 6 tablespoons raw shredded carrot, ½ cup chopped cucumber, and 2 tablespoons Caesar salad dressing

Colombian Mango Dessert (page 269)

Pre- and Post-Exercise Snacks

1 energy bar or nutrition drink

Dried figs + 1 slice cheese

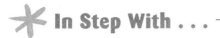

In Step With . . .

Beth Rinder, Staatsburg, New York

In the spring of 2004, Beth was diagnosed with breast cancer. She endured a double mastectomy, six months of chemotherapy, and various mini-surgeries, some of which involved breast reconstruction.

After her ordeal, Beth spent some relaxation time in Miami, Florida, where she heard about a new exercise program called Zumba. She immediately located classes in the area and started attending.

Beth had been involved in the fitness industry for many years, both as a full-time participant and a part-time instructor. But as an owner of a small business, she worked long hours, leaving little time to teach. However, after experiencing her life-altering illness and discovering Zumba Fitness, she sold her business and became a full-time Zumba instructor.

"Zumba is my passion. I teach seven Zumba classes a week here in New York," she says. "When I return to Florida for the winter, I teach Zumba classes at Ocean Reef in Key Largo. In addition, I use several Zumba techniques as a personal trainer for those clients who want something more than a trainer who watches them move from machine to machine.

"Zumba has been life-affirming as well as an avenue to achieving my own highest level of physical fitness. With Zumba rhythms flowing, I am literally dancing my way through my wonderful life."

PLANNING YOUR OWN MEALS

One of the best diet habits practiced by people who have lost weight and kept it off is meal planning, from making a shopping list to strategizing and preparing the week's breakfasts, lunches, dinners, and snacks. Also, knowing what and when you will eat helps keep you from unplanned snacking that leads to unhealthy food choices. With a plan, you will avoid impulse buys when grocery shopping. Convenience is another benefit, too. By planning your meals ahead of time, you can even prepare them on weekends and freeze them if you are too busy to cook during the week. The Zumba Meal Planner below will help you plan your meals in advance so you can shed pounds and keep them off. Above all, enjoy yourself and savor what you eat!

THE ZUMBA MEAL PLANNER

MEAL	FOODS
Date:	
Breakfast	Light Protein:
	Starch:
	Fruit:
	Beverage:
Lunch	Light Protein:
	Starch:
	High-Volume Vegetable:
	Fruit:
Dinner	Light Protein:
	Starch:
	High-Volume Vegetable:
Healthy Fat Allotment	
Pre-Exercise Snack	
Post-Exercise Snack	

Eating Out on the Zumba Diet

It is normal to want to get out of the kitchen occasionally and let someone else do the cooking for you. But what about sticking to the Zumba Diet? Will dining out strike a fatal blow to your resolve? Not necessarily. These days, most restaurants cater to health-conscious diners, so it is not that difficult to find low-fat cuisine while dining out.

You do not have to be a recluse while on the Zumba Diet. You are free to go out to restaurants, even fast-food places, to enjoy breakfast, lunch, or dinner with your friends, family, or business associates. Nor should you pass up invitations to parties or other social events just because you are on a healthy eating program.

Following are some practical guidelines for making healthy choices at any type of restaurant, as well as for enjoying parties and other events.

Choose Your Restaurant Wisely

The best restaurants to choose are those that offer a "light" or "healthy" menu and those that are willing to accommodate special requests. Whenever possible, select a restaurant that makes its meals' nutrition information available. Many chain restaurants post nutrition information on their websites. For a better idea of what to expect at the restaurant, consider calling ahead to ask questions or obtain a copy of the menu. You might be able to access the menu online.

Have It Your Way

Before ordering your selections, ask the server about the details of the meal. This will help you make more informed choices. Some questions to ask include:

* How is this dish prepared? Can it be modified?

* What ingredients are used?

* Do you have any low-fat or low-calorie options?

* What comes with this meal?

* Can I make substitutions?

* How large are the portions?

Do not be afraid to make special requests. For example, ask that foods be served with minimal butter, margarine, or oil. Ask if a particular dish can be broiled or baked rather than fried. Also, ask that no additional salt be added to your food if you are watching your sodium. You can always order dressings, sauces, or toppings on the side so that you can decide how much you actually use. Measure out a small amount of sauce or dressing with your spoon, or, with thicker salad dressing, use the fork-dipping method to coat the fork before you spear each bite. That way you get a taste with each bite of salad. You can also ask for a lower-fat or lower-calorie dressing, such as vinaigrette.

You may also be able to make substitutions. If the ingredients are on the menu, the chef should be able to accommodate your needs. A common substitution is a baked potato for fries, or a double serving of vegetables instead of a starch. If your dish does not arrive at the table the way you ordered it, do not be afraid to send it back for revisions. After all, you are paying the bill, so your food should be prepared the way you want it. Be "health assertive"!

Make a Meal Out of Appetizers

Certain appetizers can be excellent choices for an entrée. The portion size of appetizers is often more appropriate than huge portions provided in entrées. Consider healthful options such as steamed seafood (for example, shrimp cocktail), salads that are not piled high with fatty stuff (such as cheese and bacon), grilled vegetables, and broth-based soups. You might also choose to combine the appetizer with a salad; the salad will help you feel full without adding a lot of calories. Watch out for certain appetizers, however. Those that are fried or covered in cheeses, oils, and cream sauces are drenched with calories and fat.

Choose Low-Fat Preparation Methods

The way your entrée is prepared will influence the calorie and fat content. For example, grilled chicken is lower in fat and calories than fried chicken. (If you are served chicken with skin, you can remove the skin to save a ton of fat and calories.) When you choose dishes prepared with higher-fat methods, eat less of those dishes and pair the choice with a low-fat salad or vegetable to add volume for fewer calories.

Practice Portion Control

Most restaurants serve too much food—at least two to three times the quantity we need in a meal. Consider sharing a meal or taking a doggie bag so that you can have a quick meal at a later time. As you are eating, listen to your internal hunger signals and stop when you have had enough. Eating slowly helps you recognize such cues.

Now here are specific tips for different kinds of restaurants:

Restaurants for Breakfast

✳ Order scrambled egg whites, or scrambled egg substitutes (such as Egg Beaters). Request that the eggs be cooked without added oil.

✳ For carbohydrates, your best bets are oatmeal or oat bran with skim milk. Another good choice is whole-wheat or rye toast.

✳ Fresh fruits are excellent choices to round out your breakfast.

Asian Restaurants

✳ Select entrées made with lean proteins (such as chicken and fish) and vegetables. Some good suggestions for ordering are moo goo gai pan, Szechwan shrimp or chicken, and sushi.

✳ Request that the sauce be served on the side, or forgo it altogether.

✳ Asian restaurants serve generous helpings. Consider ordering one entrée and splitting it with a friend, unless you want to take the leftovers home.

Italian Restaurants

✳ For an appetizer, try vegetable antipasto (if available), with dressing on the side.

✳ Look for entrées such as grilled chicken and fish, as well as Italian dishes that are marked as low in fat.

✳ Avoid entrées prepared in cream sauce or Alfredo sauce.

- Ask the waiter to leave the rolls and breadsticks in the kitchen.

- When ordering a dinner salad, request dressing on the side.

- Opt for steamed vegetables as your side dish over pasta. Make sure the vegetables are steamed rather than cooked in fats or prepared another unhealthy way.

Mexican Restaurants

- Grilled chicken, shrimp, or lean-meat entrées are good choices.

- Request *pico de gallo* (a mixture of chopped tomatoes, green peppers, and onions).

- Mexican rice or black bean soup are nice accompaniments to a Mexican meal.

- A dinner salad with nonfat salad dressing is a healthy meal-starter.

Steakhouses

- Order grilled lean meat, chicken, salmon, or other fish (prepared without oil).

- For a side dish, select a steamed vegetable such as broccoli.

- At the salad bar, stick to fresh vegetables and nonfat or low-fat salad dressing. Many salad bars serve fresh fruit, too, which makes for a great dessert.

Homestyle or Cafeteria Restaurants

- Request grilled or lemon chicken, turkey breast without the gravy, or white fish prepared without sauce or oil.

- Select steamed vegetables (no sauce or butter), salad with nonfat dressing, or carrot/vegetable medley prepared without butter or margarine.

- Blindfold yourself when passing by the dessert line.

Delis

- A good protein choice is sliced turkey or chicken breast.

- Request that your sandwich be prepared on whole-grain bread.

* Order steamed-vegetable side dishes, if available, or a plain salad with reduced-fat dressing.

* Request that your sandwich be prepared with mustard only, to save on fat.

Fast-Food Restaurants

* Most fast-food establishments have salads on their menus; grilled chicken salads are your best bets. Order reduced-fat salad dressing with your salad. If there is a salad bar, stick to fresh vegetables and fat-free salad dressing.

* At fast-food restaurants that serve fish, order baked fish, steamed vegetables, and a salad.

Parties

* Eat a meal before you go to the party to fend off hunger pangs and cravings.

* Snack on fresh vegetables and fruit (but pass up the dip).

* If you are going to dinner with a group of friends and are concerned that you'll overeat, eat some natural high-fiber foods (like raw vegetables or fruit) before you go. You will be less likely to overindulge later.

* Offer to bring a couple of your own dishes (low fat, of course) to the gathering.

* Instead of a cocktail, drink a diet soda or carbonated water with a twist of lemon or lime.

On the surface, it may not seem like fun to limit yourself to certain foods when eating out. But rest assured: The ability to make healthy choices at restaurants or social events is just one more positive step toward getting in super-shape. You will feel better, and your body will love you for it.

Chapter 12
THE ZUMBA DIET RECIPES

The Zumba Diet recipes give you a delicious way to reach your weight-loss goals and energize you for Zumba and other exercises. Each recipe has been created to help you succeed at getting your weight under control, without skimping on the flavors you love.

Lots of care has been taken to make sure this batch of recipes is easy to follow and simple to prepare. There are no long lists of ingredients, complicated cooking methods, or hard-to-understand directions. The Zumba Diet recipes require no special equipment, either, although some appliances can make food preparation easier, such as a blender and a microwave oven. Barely know how to boil water? Wouldn't have a clue what to do with a stewpot? Good news. You do not even have to be a good cook to prepare these recipes! And all the recipes are built around foods you can buy at the grocery store.

There is a wide variety of recipes here, too. Pizza, fried chicken, lasagna, and cheesecake hardly sound like part of a dream diet. Yet foods like these are all here and are sure to satisfy your taste buds. We have even tossed in several classic Colombian dishes to give you a taste of the culture! Regardless of the plan you follow—the Zumba Basic Diet, the Zumba Flat Abs Diet, and the Zumba Thin Thighs Diet—you can use any of these recipes. But if you are following the thigh or abs plan, you can easily figure out which recipes are best for you by checking the listed ingredients for bodyshaping foods.

The Zumba Diet recipes are low in fat and calories, made leaner and healthier by using cooking methods such as broiling, steaming, baking, lightly stir-frying, microwaving, and sautéing in water or with nonstick spray. When the recipes do call for oil, it is always a healthy oil. With every new recipe you try, you learn low-fat and low-carb cooking tips; healthy methods of food preparation; ways to cut the fat, sugar, and calories; and how to use fresh herbs and spices, onions, peppers, garlic, and leeks to add flavor when you cut back on fat and salt. Plus, our recipes show you what a cinch it is to prepare healthy starches and whole grains in a nutritious way.

Some of the recipes make just one serving. If others in your household are following the Zumba Diet, you can easily make these single-serve recipes in extra quantities. Other recipes feature multiple servings. Any leftovers can be refrigerated or frozen. That way, you can defrost and/or reheat in the microwave for a quick, healthy meal.

And speaking of quick, time-savers are built into each recipe, too. For example, they take advantage of healthy convenience foods, such as boneless, skinless chicken breasts that are already pounded and cut up, prewashed greens and salad mixes, and quality convenience products such as prepared salad dressings or salsas, low-calorie soups, and canned or frozen vegetables.

Once you get the hang of healthy low-calorie cooking, expect to lose your taste for greasy, sugary foods. Why? Because tastes are learned. Just as you learned to like fattening, sugary, or salty foods, your taste buds can be retrained to enjoy fresh, delicious, and healthy dishes. For example, it is possible to retrain your taste buds by using herbs and spices. Salt-free seasoning blends are a good way to help yourself get out of the habit of sprinkling salt on everything. Your taste buds do adapt to what you eat.

These recipes cut unhealthy fat and calories by substituting low-calorie ingredients for high-calorie ones. You can do the same in your own cooking. Most of us use the same twelve to fifteen recipes most of the time. By tweaking them to reduce calories and fat, we can further increase our success in changing our eating habits as part of overall lifestyle changes to improve our health. Here are some examples of the changes you can make in your favorite recipes to create healthier, more nutritious dishes:

✳ **Dairy Products.** If a recipe calls for dairy products, you can always use low-fat and occasionally fat-free substitutions. For example, if it uses one cup of regular sour cream, you can usually substitute with the low-fat version, fat-free plain yogurt, or blended low-fat cottage cheese. Low-fat sour cream also blends better into hot dishes, as the fat-free type has a high water content and may separate into clumps when added to a recipe. Fat-free sour cream has its uses, however. If you are mixing it for salad dressing or dip, it works just fine. Yogurt or silken tofu can be mixed with low-fat mayonnaise in dishes such as coleslaw, tuna, and potato salad. Fat-free cream cheese is great for making low-cal desserts like cheesecake. You can also replace whole-milk products with skim milk and nondairy milk. When a recipe calls for cream, substitute evaporated skim milk or fat-free half-and-half. Substituting soy cheese for regular cheese is another option for cutting down on the amount of saturated fat.

✳ **Meats.** When selecting ground meats, look for those 90 percent fat free or higher. These are generally more expensive per pound, but you are getting more meat for your money because less fat is incorporated in the total product. If you cook ground meat, drain excess fat after browning it. Simply place a paper towel in a colander and pour the browned meat in so the towel can absorb the fat.

Should a recipe call for a high-fat meat such as bacon, you can reduce the fat by 50 to 60 percent by using bacon bits to impart the flavor. Another trick is to replace high-fat meats like pepperoni with turkey bacon or turkey pepperoni.

✳ **Bad Fats.** You can reduce or eliminate fats in recipes. For example, when sautéing or frying, simply coat nonstick pans with a spritz of vegetable oil cooking spray (0 calories) rather than using vegetable shortening or butter. Replace butter or margarine with butter-flavor sprinkles or fat-free squeeze or tub margarine that is trans-fat free. Reduce fat by one-fourth to one-third in baked goods. For example, if a recipe calls for 1 cup oil, try ½–²/₃ cup instead.

Always use high-flavor ingredients, like fresh herbs, zesty spices, and seasonal fruit, to invigorate dishes, rather than gobs of butter to add flavor. Employ clever cooking techniques, too. Our cereal-coated chicken thighs, for example, skip the plunge in hot oil and get baked instead. The result is moist, tender meat under a savory, golden crust (without the grease)—not a bad trade-off. Talk about a painless way to lose weight!

Another tip: Buy an oil mister at a kitchen or housewares store (Misto is one popular brand). You simply pour oil, such as canola or olive, into the spray bottle and then spray a fine mist of the oil over the pan or the food. This process cuts the amount of oil that you use drastically, thus reducing the calories from fat.

✳ **Desserts.** Fruit makes a great dessert but by itself may be boring to eat. Try dressing up a bowl of strawberries with either low-fat whipped cream or fat-free chocolate syrup or both. Also, you can easily redesign your favorite dessert recipes to yield less sugar, fat, and calories by switching to lower-fat ingredients and learning how to cook with lower-calorie sweeteners.

✳ **Salt.** Start by using half the amount called for in the recipe. Continue to reduce the amount until you find the minimal amount needed to season the recipe. Or replace the salt with lemon or lime juice, flavored vinegar, fresh onion or garlic, onion or garlic powder, pepper, chili powder, ginger, or other herb-only seasonings. Use low-sodium soy sauce or hot mustard sauce to replace regular soy sauce. Season food with spices and herbs as an alternative to adding salt.

As part of retraining your food habits, I encourage you to try several new recipes a week. Learning new dishes, in addition to re-creating copies of existing ones, is a great strategy for losing weight and keeping it off.

Eating should be fun! Your motivation to lose weight and keep it off will be greater when you enjoy your food, which is why learning how to prepare great-tasting yet healthy food gives you a tremendous advantage. Healthy, low-calorie cooking does not need to be bland or boring, nor must you sacrifice flavor and taste.

I hope you love what we have cooked up here. These are recipes that can satisfy your appetite and help you drop pounds.

Now—the Zumba Diet recipes. Enjoy!

BREAKFAST RECIPES

LOW-FAT, LOW-SUGAR GRANOLA

2 ½ cups apple juice

½ cup reduced-calorie syrup
(fructose-sweetened)

2 teaspoons vanilla

14 cups rolled oats

1 package dried figs, cut in pieces

2 tablespoons cinnamon

2 teaspoons nutmeg

Vegetable cooking spray

In a large saucepan, heat apple juice, syrup, and vanilla to boiling, then remove from heat. Stir in oats and figs and moisten thoroughly. Mix in cinnamon and nutmeg.

Spray three cookie sheets with vegetable cooking spray. Spread oat mixture onto the sheets and spray the mixture with Pam three times to coat it. Bake in a 325-degree oven until dry and crisp—about 50 minutes. Stir the mixture frequently during baking. Remove from oven. Let cool and pack in airtight containers. The granola does not need refrigeration. Makes 14 one-cup servings.

CINNAMON RAISIN FRENCH TOAST

1 egg, beaten

2 tablespoons fat-free half-and-half

1 slice raisin bread

Vegetable cooking spray

Dash of cinnamon

Mix beaten egg with half-and-half. Dip raisin bread in mixture until soaked through. Place bread in a nonstick frying pan that has been sprayed with vegetable spray. Cook on both sides until bread is slightly brown. Sprinkle with cinnamon prior to serving. Makes 1 serving.

WESTERN OMELET

Vegetable cooking spray

4 egg whites

2 tablespoons finely chopped
green pepper

3 tablespoons finely chopped
onion

½ cup chopped cooked turkey
bacon

¼ teaspoon salt

Dash pepper

Spray skillet with vegetable cooking spray. Beat egg whites and whisk in remaining ingredients. Pour mixture into skillet with medium heat. Cook, stirring to cook evenly. Turn and cook other side. Makes 2 servings.

SOUPS, STEWS, AND CHOWDERS

WHITE BEAN SOUP

1 tablespoon olive oil

½ cup coarsely chopped onion

1 teaspoon minced garlic (about 2 large garlic cloves)

1 cup sliced carrots

1 15-ounce can white beans, rinsed and drained

1 14½-ounce can low-fat ready-to-serve chicken broth

1 4-ounce can green chilies

¼ teaspoon oregano

¼ teaspoon freshly ground black pepper

2 cups chopped cabbage leaves

In large saucepan over medium-high heat, add to the oil the onion, garlic, and carrots. Sauté, stirring occasionally until the onion is tender, about 5 minutes. Add beans, chicken broth, chilies (undrained), oregano, and black pepper. Bring to a boil. Reduce heat and simmer, covered, for 10 minutes. Add cabbage. Cook, covered, until cabbage is crisp-tender, about 5 minutes. Serve hot. Makes 7 cups or 4 servings.

SPICY TOMATO SOUP

2 tablespoons olive oil

3 medium leeks, sliced up to the green parts

1 tablespoon minced garlic

½ teaspoon salt

14-ounce can diced tomatoes

3 cups low-sodium vegetable juice

1 teaspoon dried marjoram

¼ teaspoon fresh ground pepper

Heat oil in a large soup pot. Sauté leeks, garlic, and salt until leeks are soft. Slowly stir in tomatoes, tomato juice, marjoram, and pepper. Cover and cook on low heat for 20 minutes. Makes 4 servings.

GARDEN VEGETABLE SOUP

3 cups cabbage, chopped

2 yellow squashes, chopped

1 large onion, chopped

3 large celery stalks with leaves, chopped

2 15-ounce cans crushed tomatoes

3 14-ounce cans fat-free chicken broth

1 cup low-sodium or fresh vegetable juice

3 teaspoons salt

¼ teaspoon pepper

Place all ingredients in a large pan and simmer for one hour, or until vegetables are soft. Makes 16 servings.

AJIACO

(One of our national dishes in Colombia!)

4 chicken breasts, skin and fat removed

1 medium onion, cut into chunks

1 teaspoon minced garlic

1 medium sweet potato, cut into 8 pieces

4 cups fat-free chicken broth

6 green onions, chopped

10 sprigs fresh cilantro

2 medium Yukon Gold potatoes, peeled and thinly sliced

1 cup frozen corn, thawed

3 tablespoons capers, drained

1 cup fat-free plain yogurt

1 avocado, peeled and sliced

Place the chicken breasts, onion, garlic, yam, and broth in a large stewpot; cover and cook over low heat for 30 minutes; remove and save chicken pieces. Strain stock through a sieve: return strained stock to pot.

Add chicken, green onions, potatoes, corn, and capers to stock; simmer, covered, for 10 minutes. Remove from heat: discard cilantro sprigs. Add yogurt, stir over low heat for 1 minute.

Serve in large soup bowls. Float slices of avocado on top of each serving. Makes 4 servings.

SALMON CHOWDER

1 pound salmon fillet

½ teaspoon kosher salt

Cooking spray

¼ cup olive or canola oil

¼ teaspoon freshly ground black
   pepper

1 cup chopped onion

½ cup chopped celery

3 tablespoons cornstarch

3 cups fat-free chicken broth

2 medium potatoes, peeled and
   cut into 1-inch pieces

1 (9-ounce) package frozen corn,
   thawed

2 cups fat-free half-and-half

Preheat oven to 400 degrees. Sprinkle salmon with kosher salt and pepper. Place on a baking dish that has been sprayed with vegetable cooking spray. Bake for 15 to 20 minutes, or until fish flakes easily with a fork. Flake fish into ½-inch pieces and set aside.

Heat oil in a large saucepan over medium heat. Add onion and celery, and sauté several minutes until tender. Add cornstarch. Stir until mixture is smooth. Gradually stir in chicken broth. Cook over medium heat, stirring constantly, until thick. Add potatoes and corn and cook on low heat until potatoes are soft. Stir frequently to prevent ingredients from sticking to the bottom of the pan. Add half-and-half. Stir in salmon. Cook for 5 minutes or until entire mixture is heated throughout. Makes 4 servings.

SALADS AND SALAD DRESSINGS

ZESTY OLIVE OIL VINAIGRETTE

¼ cup white balsamic vinegar

3 tablespoons water

1 package (0.75 ounce) Good Seasons Italian or Zesty Italian salad dressing mix

½ cup olive oil

Place vinegar and water in a jar with a tight-fitting lid. Add salad dressing mix and shake vigorously until well blended. Add oil and shake again until well blended. Can be refrigerated for up to four weeks.

TUNA NICOISE SALAD

3-ounce can of tuna

½ cup cooked string beans (cold)

½ roasted red pepper, sliced

3 small boiled potatoes, sliced and chilled

Lettuce, 6 large leaves

2 tablespoons reduced-fat Italian salad dressing

In this version of the classic Nicoise salad, cauliflower can take the place of the potatoes for a lower-carb rendition. Arrange tuna, beans, and potato on a bed of lettuce. Drizzle with salad dressing. Makes 1 serving.

GOURMET SPINACH SALAD

1 ½ cups fresh spinach leaves (stems removed)

Several pieces sliced fresh mushrooms

1 oz. crumbled low-fat feta cheese (about 1½ tablespoons)

½ cup white cannelini beans, canned

1 tablespoon chopped walnuts

2 tablespoons light Raspberry Vinaigrette Salad Dressing (Light Done Right)

Arrange all ingredients on a salad plate. Drizzle with dressing. Makes 1 serving.

ARTICHOKE HEART SALAD

1 can (14 ounces) water-packed artichoke hearts, rinsed, drained, and quartered

2 medium tomatoes, diced

Red onion cut into fine rings

Zesty Olive Oil Vinaigrette

Halve artichoke hearts lengthwise; arrange, cut side up, onto two serving plates. Arrange tomato dices on artichoke heart halves. Drizzle dressing over salads and garnish plate with fine red onion rings. Refrigerate for 1 hour before serving. Makes 2 servings.

GREEK BARLEY SALAD

2 cups low-fat chicken broth, canned

1 cup barley

1 small can chopped black olives

¼ cup finely chopped red onion

1 medium tomato, diced

¼ cup cucumber, diced

Zesty Olive Oil Vinaigrette

Bring the broth to a boil in a medium saucepan. Add the barley. Bring back to a boil, adjust heat to maintain a gentle simmer, cover, and cook until tender, about 30 minutes. Remove from the heat and let stand, covered, for 10 minutes more. Drain excess liquid, if needed. Cool.

Place olives, onions, tomatoes, and cucumber in a salad bowl. Add the barley to these ingredients and toss with Zesty Olive Oil Vinaigrette to coat. Chill for at least an hour prior to serving. Makes 4 servings.

MARINATED VEGETABLE MEDLEY

2 cucumbers, peeled, seeded, and coarsely chopped

2 yellow bell peppers, coarsely chopped

4 tomatoes, coarsely chopped

20 green olives, diced

1 cup coarsely chopped red onion

Zesty Olive Oil Vinaigrette

Combine all vegetables in a large bowl. Toss with the desired amount of vinaigrette. Chill one hour and serve. Makes 4 servings.

CALI FRUIT SLAW

1 mango, sliced into julienne strips

½ cup carrots, sliced into julienne strips

1 pound jicama, sliced into julienne strips

¼ cup chopped fresh cilantro

½ cup orange juice

Combine all ingredients in a salad bowl and refrigerate until serving. Makes 4 servings.

MARINATED GARBANZO BEAN SALAD

1 can (16 oz.) garbanzo beans, rinsed and drained

¼ cup chopped onion

1 medium red bell pepper, chopped

1 teaspoon chopped garlic

2 teaspoons fresh basil, chopped

2 teaspoons fresh oregano, chopped

Marinade:

3 tablespoons olive oil

1 tablespoon red wine vinegar

½ teaspoon salt

Mix together beans, onion, red bell pepper, garlic, basil, and oregano, and place in a medium-sized bowl. Whisk together olive oil, vinegar, and salt, and pour over bean mixture. Stir ingredients together and place in the refrigerator for at least 3 hours prior to serving. Serve over a bed of lettuce. Makes 2 servings.

SIDE DISHES

"FRIED" ZUCCHINI

2 medium zucchini

6 tablespoons fat-free half-and-half

1 egg

1 cup Italian bread crumbs

¼ teaspoon Kosher salt (optional)

½ teaspoon fresh ground pepper

5 tablespoons grated Parmesan cheese

Olive oil cooking spray

Fat-free marinara sauce for dipping

Preheat oven to 425 degrees. Liberally spray a rimmed baking sheet with olive oil cooking spray. Cut zucchini in half lengthwise and if the seeds are large, scoop out seeds and discard. Cut the zucchini into French fry–type strips. In a bowl, whisk eggs and half-and-half. In a shallow dish, mix together bread crumbs, salt, pepper, and cheese. Dip the zucchini strips into the egg mixture until well coated. Roll the zucchini strips in the bread crumb mixture until well coated.

Place the strips on the baking sheet, leaving space between each piece. Spray the pieces with cooking spray. Bake for 15 minutes, or until brown. Serve with warm marinara sauce. Makes 4 servings.

GREEN BEAN CASSEROLE

1 can (10.75 oz.) low-fat condensed cream of mushroom soup

¼ cup skim milk

1 teaspoon soy sauce

¼ teaspoon fresh ground pepper

2 14.5-oz. cans French-style green beans, drained

3 tablespoons bacon bits or chips

1 medium onion, chopped

1 tablespoon olive oil

In a 1½-quart casserole dish, combine soup, milk, soy sauce, and pepper. Mix well. Add beans. Sprinkle bacon bits over the casserole.

In a small saucepan, cook onion in olive oil on high heat, until onion is brown. Place browned onions over the top of the casserole.

Bake at 350 degrees for 25 minutes.

TWICE-BAKED GARLIC CHEESE POTATOES

2 medium russet baking potatoes

2 slices turkey bacon

½ teaspoon kosher salt

½ cup cheddar cheese, shredded

¼ cup fat-free half-and-half

1 teaspoon minced garlic

¼ teaspoon fresh coarse ground black pepper

¼ cup fat-free yogurt

2 finely chopped green onions

Preheat oven to 350 degrees. Bake potatoes in preheated oven for 1 hour. Meanwhile, place bacon in a large, deep skillet. Cook over medium-high heat until evenly brown. Drain, crumble, and set aside.

When potatoes are done, let them cool for 10 minutes. Slice potatoes in half lengthwise and scoop the flesh into a large bowl; save skins. To the potato flesh, add salt, ¼ cup of the cheese, half-and-half, garlic, pepper, and yogurt. Mix with a hand mixer until well blended and creamy. Spoon the mixture into the potato skins. Top each with remaining cheese, green onions, and bacon. Bake for another 15 minutes. Makes 4 servings.

SWEET POTATO FRUIT PURÉE

2 pounds sweet potatoes, peeled
and cut into ½-inch cubes

Peel and juice of 1 large orange

1 cinnamon stick

½ cup water

1 medium apple, peeled, cored,
and chopped into ¼-inch cubes

1 banana, peeled and sliced

1 cup fat-free half-and-half

½ teaspoon nutmeg

Place the sweet potato cubes in a large pot. Add enough water to cover by 1 inch, half of the orange peel, and cinnamon stick. Bring to a boil and simmer 25 to 30 minutes or until potatoes are tender.

While the potatoes are cooking, place the fruit and the rest of the orange peel in a small saucepan with ½ cup of water and cook over medium heat, about 10 minutes. Transfer the fruit to a plate with a slotted spoon. Cook the orange juice in a small saucepan until reduced to about 1 tablespoon. Add the half-and-half and heat for about 3 minutes. Add the fruit, mix well, and simmer for another 3 minutes. Remove from heat and discard the orange peel.

When the sweet potatoes are done, drain them and discard the orange peel and cinnamon stick. Transfer the sweet potatoes to a blender and purée them. Add the fruit and nutmeg and purée again. Pour mixture into a baking dish and keep warm. Makes 6 servings.

COCONUT RICE (*ARROZ CON COCO*)

1 cup brown rice (instant)

1 tablespoon olive oil

1 teaspoon kosher salt

1 cup fat-free chicken broth

1 cup unsweetened coconut milk

1 (3-inch) cinnamon stick

Combine the rice, olive oil, salt, broth, coconut milk, and cinnamon stick in a saucepan and bring to a boil. Cover and boil gently for 15 to 20 minutes or until rice is fluffy and has absorbed all liquid. Discard cinnamon stick and fluff with a fork. As a side dish, this delicious rice can be served with grilled meats or fish. Makes 4 servings.

DILLED RICE

1 cup brown rice, uncooked

2 cups water

2 tablespoons dried dill weed

Salt

Bring rice and water to a boil. Reduce heat and simmer for 45 minutes until rice is cooked. Halfway through cooking, add dill and salt to taste. Makes 4 servings.

SOUTHWESTERN LETTUCE WRAPS

1 can black beans, drained

1 cup corn

¼ cup chopped onion

1 shredded carrot

1 jalapeno pepper, chopped (optional)

Light ranch dressing

8 large, firm lettuce leaves

Heat the beans and corn together until just warm. Carefully fill each side of a lettuce leaf with some of the bean-and-corn mixture, as you would if you were making a taco. Add a little onion, carrot, and jalapeno. Spoon on a few teaspoons of dressing. Next, roll over once, then fold each end toward the center. Finish folding the lettuce leaf by rolling it shut. Repeat this process for each wrap. Makes 8 wraps.

ENTRÉES

QUICK-FIX FAJITAS

2 low-carb flour tortillas

Strips of grilled chicken

Assorted chopped vegetables: tomatoes, green peppers, onion, jalapeno, lettuce

2 ounces reduced-fat cheddar cheese

2 tablespoons salsa

Fill tortillas with chicken, vegetables, cheese, and salsa. Fold over. Makes 2 tortillas.

ANN'S EASY CHICKEN

4 6-oz. chicken breasts

½ cup Worcestershire sauce

½ cup light soy sauce

Mix together Worcestershire sauce and soy sauce. Pour over chicken and let marinate in the refrigerator for at least 1 hour. Grill over a moderate flame, basting occasionally with the marinade. Makes 4 servings.

SAUCY SALMON

1 pound fresh salmon fillet

Cooking spray

1 (7.6-ounce) jar hoisin sauce

1 tablespoon grated orange rind

½ cup fresh-squeezed orange juice

2 tablespoons rice vinegar

1 teaspoon fresh grated ginger

½ teaspoon garlic powder

Preheat oven to 400 degrees. Cut salmon into 4 equal pieces. Spray a baking pan with cooking spray. Place fillets in pan. Spray fillets lightly with cooking spray. Bake 20 to 25 minutes, or until fish flakes easily with a fork.

In the meantime, combine hoisin sauce, grated orange rind, orange juice, vinegar, ginger, and garlic in a medium saucepan. Stir well. Cook over medium heat 5 minutes or until thoroughly heated. Spoon over baked salmon. Makes 4 servings.

EASIEST SALMON EVER

1 pound fresh salmon fillet

Old Bay Seasoning

Vegetable cooking spray

Preheat oven to 400 degrees. Cut salmon into 4 equal pieces. Spray a baking pan with cooking spray. Place fillets in pan. Sprinkle Old Bay Seasoning over fillets. Spray fillets lightly with cooking spray. Bake 20 to 25 minutes, or until fish flakes easily with a fork. Makes 4 servings.

MIAMI CRAB CAKES

1 large egg, beaten

3 tablespoons reduced-fat mayonnaise

1 tablespoon finely chopped pimentos

2 tablespoons seasoned bread crumbs

1 teaspoon Old Bay Seasoning

1 tablespoon minced parsley

½ pound lump crabmeat or surimi, shredded

2 tablespoons canola oil

Combine egg, mayonnaise, pimentos, bread crumbs, Old Bay Seasoning, and parsley. Mix well. Gently fold in crabmeat. Form into 4 patties.

Heat oil in large nonstick skillet over medium heat. Fry crab cakes, 5 to 6 six minutes on each side, or until golden brown. Makes 2 servings.

SESAME FISH

1 pound orange roughy

2 tablespoons olive oil

2 tablespoons rice vinegar

2 tablespoons light soy sauce

1 teaspoon chopped garlic

2 tablespoons sesame seeds

Spray a broiler pan with vegetable cooking spray to prevent fish from sticking. Place orange roughy on the pan. Whisk together olive oil, rice vinegar, soy sauce, and garlic until well blended. Pour over fish. Sprinkle sesame seeds over fish. Broil at medium heat about eight inches away from heat for about 20 minutes or until fish flakes easily with a fork. Makes 4 servings.

TANGY CATFISH CREOLE

1 pound catfish fillets

2 cups mild or medium chunky salsa

Place fillets in a ungreased baking dish. Pour salsa over fish. Bake uncovered in a 400-degree oven for 25 minutes or until fish flakes easily with a fork. Serve over hot brown rice. Makes 4 servings.

SCALLOP KABOBS

1 pound scallops, raw

1 medium red bell pepper

1 medium green bell pepper

1 medium yellow bell pepper

8 white pearl onions

½ cup sun-dried tomato vinaigrette dressing (reduced fat)

Cut peppers into large chunks. Arrange scallops, pepper chunks, and onions on kabob skewers. Baste with vinaigrette and grill over a medium flame for about 20 minutes, brushing with remaining dressing. Makes 4 servings.

TOFU LASAGNA

½ (12-ounce) package uncooked whole-wheat lasagna noodles

1 (12-ounce) package firm tofu, crumbled

2 eggs

¼ teaspoon kosher salt

¼ teaspoon black pepper

1 teaspoon minced garlic

1 teaspoon dried oregano

1 teaspoon dried basil

½ cup grated Parmesan cheese

1 jar sugar-free or low-carb spaghetti sauce

2 cups shredded mozzarella cheese, divided in half

Preheat oven to 350 degrees. Bring a large pot of lightly salted water to a boil. Add lasagna and cook for 8 to 10 minutes or until al dente; drain.

In a medium bowl combine tofu, eggs, seasonings, garlic, 1 cup of mozzarella cheese, and Parmesan cheese.

In a 9" x 13" pan, spoon a layer of spaghetti sauce. Then add a layer of lasagna noodles. Spoon on a layer of the tofu mixture, then a layer of sauce, then a layer of noodles. Continue layering like this until you run out of ingredients, and end with sauce on top. Top with remaining mozzarella and some parsley. Bake for 45 minutes to 1 hour, or until hot and bubbly.

QUICK ROSEMARY PORK CHOPS

2 lean pork chops (about 4 to 5 oz. each), all visible fat trimmed

2 sprigs fresh rosemary (chop leaves)

1 tablespoon minced garlic

2 tablespoons olive oil

Using medium-low heat, sauté rosemary and garlic in olive oil until spices are soft. Add the pork chops. Cook well on both sides. Salt lightly before serving. Makes 2 servings.

CARNE ASADA WITH COLOMBIAN GREEN SAUCE

For the beef:

1 pound flank steak

1 cup orange juice

¼ cup olive oil

¼ cup chopped onion

¼ teaspoon kosher salt

¼ teaspoon pepper

For the sauce:

3 jalapeno peppers, seeded

¼ cup chopped green onions

2 tablespoons chopped cilantro

1 tablespoon water

1 tablespoon apple cider vinegar

1 tablespoon fresh lime juice

¼ teaspoon kosher salt

Place meat in a shallow glass dish. Combine orange juice, olive oil, onion, salt, and pepper; pour over meat. Refrigerate for up to 8 hours, turning meat several times.

In a blender, combine jalapenos, green onions, cilantro, water, vinegar, lime juice, and salt. Refrigerate until ready to serve.

Remove meat from marinade. Grill on a hot grill to desired degree of doneness, turning occasionally and basting with marinade. Slice thin and serve with sauce.

LOW-CARB PIZZA

2 pounds lean ground beef

1 cup Italian bread crumbs

1 egg

½ cup skim milk

1 teaspoon salt

½ teaspoon pepper

1½ teaspoons garlic powder

2 teaspoons oregano

Sugar-free spaghetti sauce or pizza sauce

1 cup shredded cheese

Pizza toppings such as mushrooms, green pepper, onions, etc.

In a large bowl, mix together the meat, bread crumbs, egg, milk, salt, and spices, and spread the meat out on a pizza pan that has been sprayed with vegetable cooking spray. Bake at 350 degrees for 20 to 30 minutes. Remove from the oven and drain off any grease. Spread on spaghetti or pizza sauce any pizza toppings you like. Top with cheese. Bake 10 minutes or longer until cheese melts. Makes 8 servings.

MEAT AND RICE LOAF

1 cup cooked brown and wild rice

1 pound extra-lean ground beef

1 egg, beaten

1 medium onion, chopped

1 teaspoon salt

¼ teaspoon garlic powder

½ teaspoon dry mustard

½ teaspoon ground sage

1 tablespoon Worcestershire sauce

Mix all ingredients together and form into a loaf. Bake at 350 degrees for an hour and a half. Makes four servings.

BARBECUED STEAK

2 5-ounce steaks, all visible fat trimmed

2 cups fat-free Catalina salad dressing

2 tablespoons teriyaki sauce

2 tablespoons light soy sauce

1 tablespoon barbecue sauce

To make the marinade, combine salad dressing, teriyaki sauce, light soy sauce, and barbecue sauce. Pour over steaks and let marinate for at least 3 hours in the refrigerator. Grill steaks to desired doneness, basting occasionally with marinade. Makes 2 servings.

DESSERTS

LUSCIOUS KEY LIME PIE

1 6-ounce prepared graham-cracker crust, reduced fat

16 ounces yogurt cheese (see directions)

½ cup Splenda Sugar Blend

1 tablespoon cornstarch

½ teaspoon grated key lime peel

12 fresh key limes, juiced (about ⅓ cup of juice)

1 teaspoon vanilla extract

2 eggs, slightly beaten

1½ cups Cool Whip Free whipped topping

Preheat oven to 325 degrees. Combine the yogurt cheese, Splenda, cornstarch, key lime peel, key lime juice, and vanilla extract, mixing gently with a wire whisk or fork. Stir in the eggs. Pour into prepared pie crust. Bake 50 to 55 minutes until the center is set. Cool slightly. Refrigerate for 5 hours or overnight.

Frost pie with 1½ cups Cool Whip Free. Serve chilled. Makes 8 servings.

YOGURT CHEESE

To make yogurt cheese, line a strainer with a coffee filter or white paper towel. Place the strainer over a bowl to catch the liquid. Spoon in 32 ounces of fat-free plain yogurt. Cover and refrigerate for 8 hours or overnight. Makes about 16 ounces of yogurt cheese.

COLOMBIAN MANGO DESSERT

1 cup orange juice

3 packets unflavored gelatin

5 ripe mangoes, peeled and cut into pieces

$1/3$ cup Splenda Sugar Blend

1 cup evaporated fat-free milk

8-ounce carton Cool Whip Free whipped topping

Place the orange juice in a small saucepan and sprinkle the gelatin over it. Set aside for 5 minutes. Purée the mango pieces in a blender. Transfer the mango purée to a mixing bowl. Stir in the Splenda and mix. Warm the juice and gelatin so that the gelatin dissolves completely. Stir the gelatin into the mango mixture. Fold in the whipped topping. Fill a 10-cup gelatin mold with the mango mixture. Cover with plastic wrap and refrigerate 2 to 3 hours. Makes 5 to 6 servings.

CHERRY CHEESECAKE

1 6-ounce prepared graham-cracker crust, reduced fat

2 8-ounce packages of fat-free cream cheese, softened

½ cup Splenda Sugar Blend

2 tablespoons fresh lemon juice

1 teaspoon vanilla extract

8-ounce carton Cool Whip Free whipped topping

1 can (20-ounce) sugar-free cherry pie filling

Mix together cream cheese, Splenda, lemon juice, and vanilla extract. Blend well. Fold in whipped topping. Pour mixture onto crust. Cover and refrigerate for at least 4 hours or until cheesecake is firm. Spread pie filling over the top of the cheesecake and return to the refrigerator to chill. Makes 8 servings.

SMOOTHIES

Many smoothies sold in juice shops contain added sugar and can be really huge. The largest ones can have more than 1,000 calories! But if you make your own smoothie, you can control its size, ingredients, and taste. All you need are the correct ingredients and a blender.

   The following high-nutrient, creamy shakes provide the get-up-and-go you need all day long. Drink them for breakfast, at snack time, or after a meal for dessert.

PEACHY SHAKE

1 cup skim milk

½ cup frozen peaches

¼ cup raw instant oatmeal

Combine all ingredients in a blender. Blend for about 2 minutes, until mixture is thick and smooth. Pour into a large glass and serve immediately. With the addition of oatmeal, this shake makes a delicious, complete meal. Makes 1 serving.

BERRY SOY SHAKE

1 cup frozen unsweetened blueberries

1 cup soy milk

Combine all ingredients in a blender. Blend for about 2 minutes, until mixture is thick and smooth. Pour into a large glass and serve immediately. Makes 1 serving.

TROPICAL REFRESHER

½ cup chopped mango

½ frozen banana (To make frozen bananas, peel and chop the bananas, seal in plastic bags, and place in the freezer.)

1 cup fat-free plain yogurt

Combine all ingredients in a blender. Blend for about 2 minutes, until mixture is thick and smooth. Pour into a large glass and serve immediately. Makes 1 serving.

RISE AND SHINE SMOOTHIE

2 to 3 crushed ice cubes

½ cup skim milk or nondairy milk

½ cup fat-free plain yogurt

1 teaspoon instant espresso granules

1 teaspoon unsweetened cocoa powder

1 packet artificial sweetener or 2 teaspoons sugar

Combine all ingredients in a blender. Blend for about 2 minutes, until mixture is thick and smooth. Pour into a large glass and serve immediately. Makes 1 serving.

CHOCOLATE FRAPPE

1 frozen banana, cut into bite-sized pieces

2 tablespoons sugar-free chocolate syrup

2 tablespoons creamy peanut butter

1 cup nondairy or skim milk

Combine all ingredients in a blender. Blend for about 2 minutes, until mixture is thick and smooth. Pour into a large glass and serve immediately. Makes 1 serving.

STRAWBERRY SHAKE

1 cup fresh strawberries

½ cup silken tofu

2 tablespoons maple syrup or honey

6 ice cubes

Combine all ingredients in a blender. Blend for about 2 minutes, until mixture is thick and smooth. Pour into a large glass and serve immediately. Makes 1 serving.

FINAL FELIZ

These words mean "happy ending" in Spanish. The stories I hear from people through my work with Zumba Fitness all have happy endings. Many have been changed by Zumba's approach to exercise and dance: a physically challenged woman who started to regain use of immobilized limbs, a guy who emerged from a bad depression, a woman who gets out of bed at 7 A.M. in the pouring rain to get to her Zumba class, or a mom who assumed she would always be flabby and uncoordinated, for example. Their enthusiasm and newfound confidence encourages them to try more, do more. Zumba seems to have changed lives in every way. Tears come to my eyes when I hear these stories. I never would have believed Zumba could do these things. I admit I do not understand all that has happened; all I do know is that I am grateful.

Now that you have begun Zumba, followed the diet, and are achieving your goals, you may be asking yourself if you will stick with it and keep your health on a good course. I can help you answer that question. You will stay in shape, and here is why: Maybe you have shed ten pounds, twenty pounds, fifty pounds, or more, but you have gained so much more. Not only do you have a better understanding of nutrition and fitness, you love and appreciate yourself more than ever. Zumba challenges both body *and* mind. When a fitness program does that, it engages a person at a deeper level. The fitness program becomes a lifestyle—a way of living that you do not want to abandon, ever, because you have a life-altering desire to live healthier in every way. Zumba is the ultimate mind-body-spirit synthesizer.

Now that you are looking fabulous and feeling incredible, where do you go from here? How *exactly* do you maintain that Zumba body and lifestyle? Because I like helping people out, and I like seeing them reach their goals, I would like to share a few thoughts with you about how to write your own *final feliz*.

STAY SMART ABOUT FOOD

If you have reached your weight-loss goal, you can now ease up a bit on your diet. By that I mean continue to eat the same healthy foods, but add one or two extra portions of starches or fruit or a little more protein to your food plan. A small splurge here and there is okay, too. I cheat occasionally myself. I sometimes eat junk food. I eat candy bars. And of course I love my ice cream. You really do not have to give anything up; just do not go overboard.

Stick with healthy fats, cut back on sugar, and eat more fiber from fruits, vegetables and nuts, and whole grains. Drink lots of water, at least eight glasses a day. It is not a bad idea to continue to preplan a few days' worth of healthy meals and snacks at a time and figure out the best options for any situation, even eating out. Be aware of what you are eating. In short, continue doing just what you have been doing while following the plans in this book.

I also encourage you to keep a "food diary" of what you eat each day. It can help you discover which of your eating habits is sapping or adding to your energy levels. I must stress to you that keeping such a diary should not be used as a means of criticizing yourself, but as a way of becoming aware of the best choices for your lifestyle and schedule.

Make a healthy diet a part of your life, not just for a few weeks or a few months, but forever. Begin to view nutritious foods as desirable for radiant well-being and energy. Your body is all you have; you cannot afford to have it break down.

AVOID DETOURS

Learn what triggers your craving for junk foods. For example, what were you doing when you wolfed down that entire bag of potato chips? Were you watching TV? Frantically working at your computer? Or did you have guests over? Stop and pay attention. It is really important to modify your behavior. Do not eat while watching television. Try not to linger in the coffee room if that is where the vending machines are. Determine what stresses you out so that you can avoid late-night raids on the refrigerator or snack attacks at the office.

Of course, when you are down in the dumps, the natural inclination is to reach for comfort foods such as chocolate, ice cream, milk and cookies, or chips. These foods, however, tend to be laced with sugar, fat, and salt. While temporarily deflating your negative emotions, they ultimately inflate your waistline. Try *healthy* comfort foods instead, such as grains, cereals, and lean proteins. These foods have demonstrated a mood-elevating effect in studies. A healthy diet, rich with natural foods, can positively affect your mood and outlook.

When you are depressed, you become your own worst enemy. Some symptoms of depres-

The Seven Secrets of Fit People

1 They eat a nutritious breakfast, which often includes cereal. (Eating breakfast reduces hunger pangs and possible "pigging out" at or before lunch.)

2 They follow a balanced, low-fat diet.

3 They limit portion sizes.

4 They pay attention to calories.

5 They enjoy a variety of fruits and vegetables.

6 They do 60 to 90 minutes of moderate-intensity physical activity per day.

7 They weigh themselves often.

Source: National Weight Control Registry

sion include feeling hopeless or tired, as well as having problems with sleep, appetite, concentration, and memory. Good health habits, social support, and maintaining an objective outlook are all effective coping strategies. If you do find yourself in a bad funk, pop in the Zumba DVD that accompanies this book, start moving, and you will get an immediate lift in your mood.

Life is anything but static. You never know what is going to happen. When one of life's curveballs comes along, some people throw in the towel. They stop exercising and sit on the couch eating cookies. Do not let this happen to you. If you are feeling overwhelmed about something, the best thing you can do is work your body. Doing something is always better than doing nothing, and doing nothing is never an option. Stick to the schedule you had before the curveball came.

 ## In Step With . . .

Kara Norick, Littleton, Colorado

No one knows better than Kara Norick that miscarriage is one of the most difficult life events to cope with. She has had four. She credits Zumba with helping her live through her grief.

After the miscarriage of her fourth child, Kara was deeply depressed and had dropped out of her Zumba class. Her instructor e-mailed her and asked Kara to return to class and just give it one more try.

"I did, and, cheesy as it sounds, Zumba saved my life," Kara says. "I was able to forget about my pain for an hour and just enjoy life. Soon, the fellowship I felt with the others in the class and the uplifting experience of the classes became a driving force in my life. I was able to find joy again, and for that I will be forever grateful.

"I am not saying that Zumba causes you to be immune from experiencing hard times in your life, or sadness, but it gives you something to look forward to. It offers a positive, self-assuring place that allows the boost needed to stay healthy, work out stress, and surround yourself with positive reinforcement that is needed to get you through those difficult times."

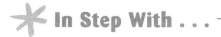

✳ In Step With . . .

Jenna Carlisle, Miami, Florida

Several years ago a hurricane struck south Florida. Jenna was getting into her car with her two children to go grocery shopping. They never made it to their destination. Suddenly, without warning, the sky darkened, and every streetlight went out. The last thing Jenna remembered was a loud crash before she blacked out.

The family was involved in a three-car pileup and was driven by three different ambulances to the hospital, lucky to be alive.

The accident was a wake-up call. Jenna knew she had to do something with her life, something that would help other people. Prior to the accident, she had been exercising at home with Zumba Fitness DVDs. Now she wanted to take it a step further by becoming a certified Zumba instructor. This was to be her calling.

Jenna has been teaching Zumba Fitness for more than two years, along with working full time at a bank and as a single mom, raising two children without the benefit of having any family around. She recently obtained an associate's degree and is working on her bachelor's degree in marketing.

"Between my full-time job, school, and my kids, sometimes I think I am going crazy, and get overwhelmed. But Zumba Fitness has helped me cope with the stress and pressure. If it weren't for Zumba, I would probably not have made it this far to where I am right now. Zumba has been the key to my success, and it has made a difference in my life!"

KEEP WEIGHT OFF EASILY WITH ZUMBA

For staying in shape, exercise is all-important. No matter what, stay faithful to your regular Zumba and exercise routine. People who manage to keep weight off exercise about 275 minutes a week, which translates to 40 minutes every day or 55 minutes five days a week, according to recent research. That is absolutely doable! If you progressed to doing five Zumba workouts a week, you would go a long way toward staying in shape, especially if you are vigilant about eating healthy foods. If you are really faithful to your diet, you may be able to get away with 30 minutes a day. If you are a little more lax, with room for some splurges, it will be closer to 60 minutes. Carve out time for Zumba every week and you will not have to struggle with your weight.

Your passion for Zumba and other physical activities is important, because it helps you look beyond the occasional sore muscle to a higher cause—getting in great shape and enjoying vibrant physical and mental health. In many ways, this calling keeps you on track. While your friends are hanging out at the mall or lounging in front of the TV, you are on a mission to transform your body into a finely tuned instrument.

CHANGE THINGS UP

It is not a good idea to let your body get used to the same workout. Always try to progress, whether that is upping the number of Zumba classes in your schedule, trying out some new DVDs, or including some yoga or other fitness activities in your week. These small tweaks will help drive your progress.

I also urge people to avoid elevators at work and hit the stairs. If you drive to work, park a few blocks away from the office and walk (if it is safe to do so). When the weather is bad, walk in the mall before or after work and on weekends. The point is to be an active person.

You should never become bored, either. Throughout the history of dance, teachers and dancers together have steadily made innovations in the way dance is taught, performed, and perceived. Zumba is no different. Change your routines so that you do not get bored. Find some new music to energize your workout. New workouts and new music will keep you excited and constantly challenged.

TUNE INTO YOUR BODY

It happens. You come back from vacation and are shocked at what you see on the scale. Sure, your weight will go up and down, but set a range that you will stay within. Establish your trigger number, such as a five-pound gain limit, and then get back into action. Resume the Zumba Diet and step up the frequency of your Zumba workouts.

For many people, weighing themselves on a regular basis helps them stay under that trigger number. "Regular" could mean every day, a few times a week, or weekly. Figure out what works best for you. Stepping on the scale daily, for example, does not work if you get discouraged easily. Just know that keeping tabs on your weight offers a way to realize your weight is creeping upward before it gets out of control. This allows you to get back on track faster with your weight loss.

KEEP YOUR PRIORITIES IN LINE

Jot down your top ten reasons for wanting to stay in shape on a note card and keep it handy at all times. Maybe you want to have more energy, not huff and puff going up the stairs, or lower your risk for some disease. Whatever motivates you to continue on your fitness journey should be put on your list. If you ever feel as if you are about to backslide, read through the list and take a few deep breaths. Step back and regroup. You will be fine. Above all, you need a reason for what you are doing.

Make yourself your own priority, too. If you are busy taking care of the family and have little time to yourself, it is tempting to let your plan slip. Many of the most successful Zumba participants have developed a healthy sense of self-centeredness: They commit to setting aside time to do things they enjoy, whether it is Zumba, getting a massage, or just having fun with their friends. So say good-bye to your guilt. Do not worry that if you always take extra time for yourself, you will be taking away from your family. The opposite is true. When you are healthy and happy, you have a lot more energy to be the spouse, partner, parent, child, or friend you want to be.

In Step With . . .

Nancy Hildebrandt, Chicago, Illinois

All her life, Nancy loved to dance but never had any formal training. So, as a way to express herself through dance, she taught dance-based group exercise classes while attending college. However, after college she decided to pursue a corporate career rather than a fitness career. Nancy remained very active throughout her twenties and into her thirties. Her life got more complicated and busier each year that followed, and exercise became more sporadic. Two decades after college and having spent too many years behind a desk, Nancy decided it was time to devote herself to fitness—and dance—on a more substantial level. Then along came Zumba.

"I had never heard of Zumba before spring 2006, when I received a random e-mail announcing there was a Zumba instructor training class coming to my town," she recalls. "After a bit of research, I realized that this was just the thing I needed to get me back on track. Even if I never taught a single Zumba class, I knew that attending this course would jump-start my return to an active lifestyle. Little did I know just how much influence Zumba would have on my life."

Nancy fell completely in love with Zumba during the training class. And she realized that fitness and dance always were truly her passion. "How incredibly fortunate I felt to have found a way to combine these two loves of my life!"

Zumba gave Nancy the confidence to leave the corporate world behind and dedicate herself full time to the business of health and fitness. After becoming licensed as a Zumba instructor, she became an AFAA-certified group exercise instructor, and is now pursuing certification as a personal trainer.

"I love helping others discover their capabilities beyond what they ever imagined they could do. I'm finally living the dream I had so many years ago, doing what I love, and I'm actually getting paid to do it! What more could a person ask for!"

EMPOWER YOURSELF

Affirmations are positive messages you tell yourself. These messages act like a pair of eye-glasses that improve vision. They help you make perceptual changes in the ways you view your body, food, eating, health, and life.

Focusing on your affirmations helps you in two ways. First, attention is drawn to the meaning of the advice and away from bad habits. Second, it allows time for your mind to internalize the message so that it becomes a part of the way you think and act.

Choose affirmations that are believable and make sense to you. Use three to four messages at a time, repeating each at different times. Here are some suggestions that you can use or edit for yourself.

I deserve to be happy, healthy, and successful.

My body is a beautiful gift that deserves to be respected and nurtured.

I have the power to make the healthiest choices for myself.

I see myself looking fit and feeling strong and healthy.

Good choices are gifts to myself.

KEEP BUILDING ON YOUR SUCCESS

Your transformation began on the outside and worked its way in. It is important to reflect on all your accomplishments, no matter how small they might seem. The best way to build self-confidence is to pay attention to what you are doing right. Each mini-milestone—say, completing three Zumba sessions this week or having just one helping of a favorite food (not two or three)—will keep you motivated and make you feel more confident in every area of your life.

Also, ask yourself: How much credit do I give myself at the end of the day? If your answer is not much, your confidence is going to suffer. My advice is to set aside time each day to list your accomplishments. You should feel a whole lot better, particularly if you keep the focus on you, versus what everyone else is doing. Confidence also depends on developing a healthy attitude toward mistakes. No one is perfect. If you approach a mistake as a problem to solve rather than a sign of failure, it will be easier to reach your potential.

Give yourself frequent pats on the back. You deserve them. Hear the praise you get from others—how trim you look, about what you are wearing, or the way you have fixed your hair. Hear and accept it. Silently agree with the praise. Agreeing with praise sends your brain a healthy message. It is another step toward building self-esteem. Self-esteem leads to self-confidence, and that leads to believing in yourself. Nothing—I mean nothing—is more useful than believing in yourself.

No matter where you are in your journey, keep going and do not give up. You can achieve whatever you want in life. Anyone can get in great shape, get healthier, and have a better life, no matter what his or her size, age, or physical condition. Everything is possible!

I hope you have had fun at my party. I will see you next time.

Zumba!

Zumba Fitness Resources

Zumba Fitness DVDs

If you want to order our Zumba Fitness DVD Collection, please visit www.zumbafitness.com or call 1-800-964-9141.

The Zumba Academy

The Zumba Academy provides many opportunities for fitness and dance instructors to learn to teach Zumba so that they can offer Zumba Classes at their facilities. First-time (new) instructors are also welcome to begin their teaching journey with Zumba. Anyone interested in teaching a Zumba course must attend a Zumba Instructor Training Workshop and then must keep their instructor status current through the many options offered by the Zumba Academy. Information on the Academy can be accessed at www.zumba.com.

Finding a Zumba Instructor

Please click on "Find a Class" in the main navigation on www.zumba.com.

Zumba Workshops

The Zumba Workshops train people to become Zumba instructors. The workshops that have been officially scheduled are posted in our Workshops section on www.zumba.com. If you don't find any Zumba Workshops currently scheduled in your area, keep checking as we update our website constantly. If you know of a facility that might be interested in hosting a Zumba Workshop, ask the potential host to contact us at:

Zumba Fitness, LLC.
3801 N 29th Ave.
Hollywood, FL 33020
954-925-3755 (Office)
954-925-3505 (Fax)

Zumbawear and Other Products

Log on to www.zumba.com and click on the "Shop" link on the navigation bar. For all other information, contact us at:

Zumba Fitness, LLC.
3801 N 29th Ave.
Hollywood, FL 33020
954-925-3755 (Office)
954-925-3505 (Fax)

References

Part One: Ditch the Workout, Join the Party!

Herzberg, G. R. 2004. Aerobic exercise, lipoproteins, and cardiovascular disease: benefits and possible risks. *Canadian Journal of Applied Physiology* 29:800–807.

Phillips, L. K., and J. B. Prins. 2008. The link between abdominal obesity and the metabolic syndrome. *Current Hypertension Reports* 10:156–164.

Poirier, P., and J. P. Despres. 2001. Exercise in weight management of obesity. *Cardiology Clinics* 19:459–470.

Salmon, P. 2001. Effects of physical exercise on anxiety, depression, and sensitivity to stress: a unifying theory. *Clinical Psychology Review* 21:33–61.

Shaw, K., et al. 2006. Exercise for overweight or obesity. *Cochrane Database of Systematic Reviews* October 18:CD003817.

Talanian, J. L., et al. 2007. Two weeks of high-intensity aerobic interval training increases the capacity for fat oxidation during exercise in women. *Journal of Applied Physiology* 102:1439–1447.

Verghese, J., et al. 2003. Leisure activities and the risk of dementia in the elderly. *New England Journal of Medicine* 348:2508–2516.

Wachi, M., et al. 2007. Recreational music-making modulates natural killer cell activity, cytokines, and mood states in corporate employees. *Medical Science Monitor* 13:CR57–70.

Winett, R. A., and R. N. Carpinelli. 2001. Potential health-related benefits of resistance training. *Preventive Medicine* 33:503–513.

Part Three: Ditch Boring Diets: Let's Eat to Burn Belly Fat and Thigh Fat!

Adam-Perrot, A., et al. 2006. Low-carbohydrate diets: nutritional and physiological aspects. *Obesity Reviews* 7:49–58.

Barbosa, J. C., et al. 1990. The relationship among adiposity, diet, and hormone concentrations in vegetarian and nonvegetarian postmenopausal women. *American Journal of Clinical Nutrition* 51:798–803.

Burton-Freeman, B. 2000. Dietary fiber and energy regulation. *Journal of Nutrition* 130: 272S–275S.

Butryn, M. L., et al. 2007. Consistent self-monitoring of weight: a key component of successful weight loss maintenance. *Obesity* 15:3091–3096.

Catenacci, V. A., et al. 2008. Physical activity patterns in the National Weight Control Registry. *Obesity* 16:153–161.

Daeninick, E., and M. Miller. 2006. What can the national weight control registry teach us? *Current Diabetes Reports* 6:401–404.

Ditschuneit, H. H., et al. 2001. Value of structured meals for weight maintenance: risk factors and long-term weight maintenance. *Obesity Research* 9: 284S–289S.

Esmaillzadeh, A., et al. 2007. Fruit and vegetable intakes, C-reactive protein, and the metabolic syndrome. *American Journal of Clinical Nutrition* 84:1489–1497.

Garaulet, M., et al. 2006. Relationship between fat cell size and number and fatty acid composition in adipose tissue from different fat depots in overweight/obese humans. *International Journal of Obesity* 30:899–905.

Halkjoer, J., et al. 2006. Intake of macronutrients as predictors of 5-year changes in waist circumference. *American Journal of Clinical Nutrition* 84:789–797.

Hays, N. P., et al. 2004. Effects of an ad libitum low-fat, high-carbohydrate diet on body weight, body composition, and fat distribution in older men and women: a randomized controlled trial. *Archives of Internal Medicine* 164:210–217.

Higgins, J. A. 2004. Resistant starch: metabolic effects and potential health benefits. *Journal of AOAC International* 87:761–768.

Higgins, J. A., et al. 2004. Resistant starch consumption promotes lipid oxidation. *Nutrition & Metabolism.* October, pp. 1–12.

Howarth, N. C., et al. 2001. Dietary fiber and weight regulation. *Nutrition Reviews* 59:129–139.

Lejeune, M. P., et al. 2005. Additional protein intake limits weight regain after weight loss in humans. *British Journal of Nutrition* 93:281–289.

Maskarinec, G., et al. Soy intake is related to a lower body mass index in adult women. *European Journal of Nutrition* 47:138–144.

Moeller, L. E., et al. 2000. Isoflavone-rich soy favorably affects regional fat and lean tissue in menopausal women. *Experimental Biology* 2000, San Diego, CA. April 15–18. Abstract 348.4, p. A487.

No authors listed. 2005. Recipe for a healthier diet. New dietary guidelines for a healthy lifestyle: eat more whole grains, fruits, vegetables, and exercise an hour or more a day. *Health News* 11:3–4.

Paniagua, J. A., et al. 2007. Monounsaturated fat-rich diet prevents central body fat distribution and decreases postprandial adiponectin expression induced by a carbohydrate-rich diet in insulin-resistant subjects. *Diabetes Care* 30:1717–1723.

Williams, P. G., et al. 2008. Cereal grains, legumes, and weight management: a comprehensive review of the scientific evidence. *Nutrition Reviews* 66:171–182.

Wing, R. R., et al. 2001. Successful weight loss maintenance. *Annual Review of Nutrition* 21: 323–341.

Wyatt, H. R., et al. 2002. Long-term weight loss and breakfast in subjects in the National Weight Control Registry. *Obesity Research* 10:78–82.

Zemel, M. B. 2005. The role of dairy foods in weight management. *Journal of the American College of Nutrition* 24(6 Suppl.):537S–546S.

Zemel, M. B., et al. 2005. Dairy augmentation of total and central fat loss in obese subjects. *International Journal of Obesity* 29:391–397.

About the Authors

Alberto "Beto" Perez is the creative genius behind Zumba, the fitness formula that has revolutionized the way millions of people think about exercise. Beto began as a fitness instructor in his home city of Cali, Colombia. One day, upon arriving to one of his classes, he realized he had left his traditional aerobics music at home. Improvising, he unpacked some salsa and merengue tapes from his backpack, popped them into the sound system, and taught his first Zumba class!

After a relatively successful career as a trainer and choreographer in Colombia, Beto decided to make the big move to the United States. Armed only with his personal charisma and unstoppable will power, he sold all his belongings and moved to Miami in search of the American Dream. He didn't speak a word of English.

At first, Beto had a rough time settling in to his new environment, but due to his relentless dedication, he managed to quickly surpass this period of hardship. After several months, his talent and magnetism landed him a job as an instructor at a prestigious local health club. Not surprisingly, with his catchy, danceable aerobic routines performed to the tune of upbeat Latin rhythms, Beto's ZUMBA class soon became the most popular at the gym—just as had occurred in his native Colombia! He also became renowned for his sincere passion for making people enjoy their workout, consequently improving their lifestyles.

In 2001, his innovative style caught the attention of two entrepreneurs: Alberto Perlman and Alberto Aghion. Instinctively seeing Zumba's enormous business potential, they wasted no time in teaming up with Beto to create Zumba Fitness, LLC. With Beto's help, the company's current CEO and COO, respectively, have since turned Zumba into a worldwide movement. Today, Zumba is one of the largest fitness programs in the world, with millions of DVD's sold, and some 30,000 Zumba Fitness instructors in over thirty-five countries.

Why? Because it's the best party around.

Maggie Greenwood-Robinson, PhD, is a leading health and medical writer in the United States. She has authored or coauthored more than forty books on nutrition, exercise, weight loss, brain fitness, and health issues such as cancer. She is also the best-selling author of *The Biggest Loser, The Biggest Loser Fitness Plan,* and *The Biggest Loser Success Secrets,* (three of the official diet/fitness books for the NBC hit reality show).